Anesthesiology Demystified for the Internist

Aibek Mirrakhimov

Anesthesiology Demystified for the Internist

Core Concepts in Perioperative Decision-Making

Springer

Aibek Mirrakhimov
Department of Anesthesiology, Perioperative,
Critical Care, and Pain Medicine
University of Kentucky
Lexington, KY, USA

ISBN 978-3-032-16810-8 ISBN 978-3-032-16811-5 (eBook)
https://doi.org/10.1007/978-3-032-16811-5

This Springer imprint is published by the registered company Springer Nature Switzerland AG
The registered company address is: Gewerbestrasse 11, 6330 Cham, Switzerland

I dedicate this book to the memory of my grandparents, who showed me the enduring power of love, hard work, and a steadfast moral compass.

To my parents, for their unwavering support and for always being by my side when I needed it most.

To my children, Demir and Sofia, to my wife Aziza, and to our four-legged son Spark—you mean the world to me and the reason I look forward to coming home each day.

To my brother Rustam and his family, whose encouragement and companionship I deeply treasure.

To our patients, who place their trust in us—the greatest honor and privilege of this profession

And to my mentors, teachers, and colleagues, who have shaped me and taught me more than they may ever realize.

Foreword

It is a great pleasure to introduce *Anesthesiology Demystified for the Internist: Core Concepts in Perioperative Decision-Making*, authored by Dr. Aibek Mirrakhimov. In this unique and timely work, Dr. Mirrakhimov bridges two intellectually demanding disciplines in medicine: Internal Medicine and Anesthesiology.

Dr. Mirrakhimov is exceptionally qualified to undertake this endeavor. He is trained and board certified in Internal Medicine, Critical Care Medicine, Anesthesiology, and Adult Cardiac Anesthesiology, and additionally holds certifications in Advanced Perioperative Transesophageal Echocardiography, Critical Care Echocardiography, and Adult Echocardiography. His academic appointment in the Department of Anesthesiology, Perioperative, Critical Care, and Pain Medicine at the University of Kentucky reflects his dedication to clinical excellence, education, and interdisciplinary collaboration. Few physicians are as uniquely positioned to interpret perioperative physiology through both the internist's and the anesthesiologist's lenses.

This book addresses an increasingly recognized need in modern medicine, which is the integration of perioperative knowledge across specialties. Internists, hospitalists, and subspecialists are often tasked with preoperative optimization, postoperative co-management, and complex consultative decisions. Yet the language, priorities, and physiology of anesthesia can seem opaque to those outside the operating room. This book succeeds in making these principles accessible, clinically relevant, and immediately applicable to patient care.

What distinguishes this book is its emphasis on decision-making. Rather than merely describing anesthetic techniques, it explores why specific choices are made, the underlying physiologic trade-offs, and how understanding these decisions can enhance interprofessional communication and improve patient outcomes.

The text is logically organized. Part I introduces readers to the origins and structure of anesthesiology, emphasizing why internists benefit from understanding its scope. Parts II–IV explore the perioperative environment, basics of anesthetic pharmacology, and monitoring from core physiological foundations to practical applications across diverse procedural settings. Part V provides an invaluable overview of common postoperative complications, including major cardiac, pulmonary, renal, hepatic, hematologic, and neurologic, each discussed with clarity and evidence. Finally, Part VI brings these elements together through perioperative consultation frameworks, case-based scenarios, and a forward-looking discussion of how perioperative medicine is evolving into a truly collaborative specialty.

In an era where multidisciplinary care defines quality and safety, Dr. Mirrakhimov's work exemplifies the collaborative spirit that advances our field. I am confident that this book will become an indispensable resource for trainees and practicing clinicians alike.

Zaki U. Hassan

Professor and Chair
Department of Anesthesiology,
Perioperative, Critical Care,
and Pain Medicine University of Kentucky
Lexington, KY, USA

Preface

One of the central goals of this book is not to replace conversations with anesthesiologists but to enhance the quality of collaboration between anesthesiology and internal medicine. This book is written for general internists, hospitalists, and internal medicine subspecialists who frequently participate in perioperative care yet often lack structured exposure to the principles and practice of anesthesiology.

It is important to emphasize that this work is by no means a comprehensive textbook of anesthesiology. Rather, it is designed to serve as a bridge—a resource that supplements existing perioperative texts by educating internists on the nuances of anesthesia care and the reasoning that underpins anesthetic decision-making. The ultimate aim is to improve communication, foster trust, and empower internists to engage more effectively with anesthesia colleagues.

Internal medicine and anesthesiology are, at their core, disciplines of collaboration. Nowhere is this more evident than in the perioperative environment, where internists, anesthesiologists, surgeons, nurses, and allied professionals come together to care for patients at their most vulnerable.

As someone who has had the privilege of being trained and board certified in both internal medicine and anesthesiology, I have witnessed both the tremendous potential and the occasional gaps in communication between these two vital specialties.

My journey began in internal medicine and critical care, where I learned the art of longitudinal patient care, risk stratification, and the management of complex comorbidities across acute and chronic illnesses. Later, I pursued residency and fellowship in general anesthesiology and adult cardiac anesthesiology, ultimately achieving board certification in both. Alongside these, I obtained credentials in advanced perioperative transesophageal echocardiography, critical care echocardiography, and adult echocardiography, which have enriched my understanding at the intersection of diagnostics, perioperative physiology, and acute decision-making. This dual perspective has shaped my career and informs every page of this book.

Internists frequently intersect with anesthesiology in daily practice, whether through preoperative consultations, managing patients in the ICU, or co-managing perioperative complications. Yet formal exposure to anesthesiology during internal medicine training remains limited. Many internists therefore approach perioperative discussions with incomplete insight into anesthesia's scope, the nuances of anesthetic techniques, or the reasons behind intraoperative decisions. This knowledge gap can hinder collaboration, delay decision-making, and at times compromise patient safety.

The goal of *Anesthesiology Demystified for the Internist: Core Concepts in Perioperative Decision-Making* is to bridge that gap. This book introduces internists to the history and structure of anesthesiology, the dynamics of the operating room and nonoperating room environments, the pharmacology of commonly used anesthetic agents, and the core types of anesthesia, from monitored anesthesia care to neuraxial, regional, and general techniques. It also highlights areas of special relevance to internists: post-anesthesia recovery, perioperative complications, postoperative pain, and crisis management.

Equally important are the sections that focus on patient safety, perioperative medicine, and interprofessional collaboration. Anesthesiology has been a pioneer in safety science, introducing checklists, crisis resource management, and standardized monitoring long before these became universal in medicine.

This book is not intended to make internists into anesthesiologists. Rather, it is meant to demystify anesthesiology: to explain why certain intraoperative choices are made, what risks different anesthetic techniques carry, and how internists can meaningfully contribute to patient optimization before surgery and to safe recovery afterward. By understanding anesthesiology's principles, internists will be better equipped to collaborate, anticipate complications, and advocate for patients in high-stakes perioperative environments. Though primarily intended for internists and internal medicine subspecialists, this book can also be a valuable resource for clinicians from other medical and surgical specialties seeking to understand the fundamental principles of anesthesiology and perioperative decision-making.

It is my hope that this book serves as a practical and approachable resource for internists, illuminating the anesthesiologist's role, clarifying shared responsibilities, and inspiring a spirit of collaboration that benefits our patients above all else.

Lexington, KY, USA Aibek Mirrakhimov

Acknowledgments

I would like to thank all my mentors and teachers who have helped shape my career and guided me to where I am today. In particular, I am deeply grateful to Dr. Zaki U. Hassan, Chair of the Department of Anesthesiology at the University of Kentucky, for his continued support and mentorship. I also extend special thanks to the Springer Medical Publishing team—Gregory Sutorius and Nishanthini Vetrivel—for their invaluable assistance with manuscript preparation.

Contents

Part I

Origins and Structure of Anesthesiology

Brief History of Anesthesia Worldwide and in the United States: From Ether to the Modern Era

1

1.1 Introduction

The history of anesthesia represents one of the most transformative chapters in the story of modern medicine. Before the introduction of anesthetic agents, surgery was often a brutal and desperate undertaking, constrained by the limits of human suffering and the surgeon's speed. The ability to render a patient insensible to pain, while simultaneously maintaining physiologic stability, revolutionized surgical practice and laid the foundation for specialties such as anesthesiology, critical care medicine, and perioperative medicine.

This chapter traces the evolution of anesthesia from its earliest roots in antiquity, through the landmark discovery of ether anesthesia in the nineteenth century, and onward to the global development of anesthesiology as a recognized medical specialty. It concludes with an emphasis on the United States, where anesthesia matured into a field that now encompasses perioperative medicine, patient safety, pain management, and critical care.

1.2 Early Concepts of Pain Relief and Sedation

Pain control in antiquity relied heavily on herbal remedies (such as opium, cannabis, etc.), alcohol, and physical methods of restraint. Ancient civilizations used opium (derived from the poppy plant), cannabis, and other botanicals with sedative properties. The Sumerians described opium as the "joy plant" as early as 3400 BCE, while Egyptian papyri and Greco-Roman texts recorded its use for surgical procedures and labor.

By the Middle Ages, combinations of alcohol, plant extracts, and hypnosis were common. "Soporific sponges," soaked in opium, mandrake, or hashish, were pressed over the patient's face before surgery. Despite these efforts, the relief was inconsistent, and mortality from shock, blood loss, and infection remained high.

A. Mirrakhimov, *Anesthesiology Demystified for the Internist*,
https://doi.org/10.1007/978-3-032-16811-5_1

1.3 The Advent of Inhalational Anesthesia

1.3.1 Nitrous Oxide

The first inhaled anesthetic discovered was nitrous oxide, synthesized by Joseph Priestley in 1772 and later popularized by Humphry Davy in the early nineteenth century. Davy noted its analgesic effects and suggested its potential for surgery, though it was initially used as a recreational "laughing gas." In 1844, dentist Horace Wells attempted to use nitrous oxide for tooth extraction in Boston. The demonstration failed, but his insight was correct. Nitrous oxide would later become a mainstay of dental and surgical anesthesia. A monument to Horace Wells is shown in Image 1.1.

1.3.2 Ether

The defining moment in anesthesia's history came on October 16, 1846, when dentist William T. G. Morton successfully demonstrated the use of ether anesthesia at Massachusetts General Hospital during the removal of a neck tumor. This "Ether Day" is often marked as the birth of modern anesthesia. News of the demonstration spread rapidly, and ether was soon adopted worldwide for surgical operations. The first demonstration of surgical anesthesia by William T.G. Morton is shown in Image 1.2.

1.3.3 Chloroform

Shortly after ether, chloroform was introduced into practice by James Young Simpson in 1847. Its rapid onset and pleasant odor made it appealing, though later

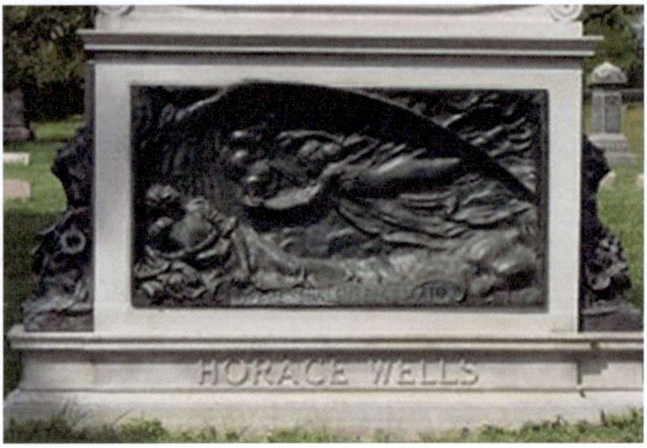

Image 1.1 Horace Wells Monument, Cedar Hill Cemetery, Hartford, CT. (Reproduced with permission from Cedar Hill Cemetery and Foundation)

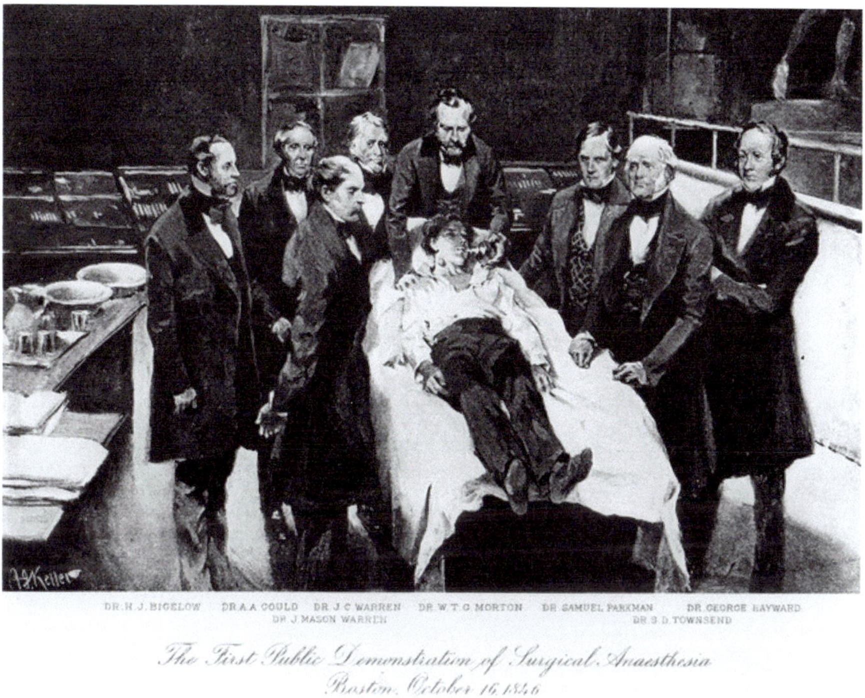

Image 1.2 The first demonstration of surgical anesthesia by William T.G. Morton. (Reproduced from https://wellcomecollection.org/works/n8j9k5cg/items under the Creative Commons Attribution 4.0 International)

recognition of hepatotoxicity and sudden cardiac death limited its long-term use. Nevertheless, chloroform gained fame when Queen Victoria received it for the birth of her eighth child in 1853, helping normalize anesthesia in obstetrics.

1.4 Growth of Anesthesia in the Nineteenth and Early Twentieth Centuries

The rapid adoption of anesthetics coincided with other innovations that reshaped surgery, including antisepsis and the development of surgical techniques requiring prolonged operating times. The ability to maintain unconsciousness expanded the scope of operations to thoracic and abdominal cavities, which were previously avoided due to pain and mortality.

By the late nineteenth century, anesthetists were increasingly recognized as essential team members. Still, anesthesia was often delivered by surgeons, medical students, or nurses, rather than dedicated specialists. The lack of formal training or standardized techniques led to variable outcomes, and anesthesia was sometimes dismissed as a "technical" rather than a medical discipline.

1.5 The Emergence of Anesthesiology as a Specialty

1.5.1 Intravenous Agents

The introduction of intravenous anesthetics marked another turning point. Barbiturates such as hexobarbital and thiopental allowed for smooth, rapid induction. Later agents, including benzodiazepines, ketamine, etomidate, and propofol, expanded the range of induction and maintenance options.

1.5.2 Muscle Relaxants and the Curare Revolution

Perhaps no single pharmacologic advance reshaped anesthesiology more profoundly than the introduction of neuromuscular blocking agents, beginning with curare. Indigenous peoples of South America had long used curare, derived from the bark and roots of *Chondrodendron tomentosum* and related plants, as a paralyzing arrow poison. Its transition from poison to medicine occurred in the twentieth century, when Canadian anesthesiologist Harold Griffith and his colleague Enid Johnson administered purified curare (intocostrin) to a patient undergoing appendectomy in Montreal in 1942.

This landmark case demonstrated that profound muscle relaxation could be achieved safely under anesthesia. Surgeons were suddenly free to operate in the abdomen and thorax without relying solely on dangerously deep levels of ether or chloroform for immobility. Anesthesiologists gained unprecedented control over the airway, enabling reliable endotracheal intubation and mechanical ventilation.

The curare revolution transformed anesthesiology from the art of keeping patients insensible to pain into a sophisticated science of pharmacologic control of consciousness, analgesia, and muscle tone. It also heralded the need for new monitoring and safety standards, as paralysis without adequate anesthesia carried the risk of catastrophic awareness and suffering.

Over the decades, synthetic and semi-synthetic neuromuscular blockers replaced crude curare preparations, offering more predictable pharmacokinetics, fewer side effects, and reversibility with anticholinesterases. Today, succinylcholine, rocuronium, vecuronium, and cisatracurium are widely used, with sugammadex providing targeted reversal of aminosteroid relaxants (see Chap. 11 for more information).

1.5.3 Monitoring and Safety

The mid-twentieth century also saw the gradual introduction of monitoring technologies. Pulse oximetry, capnography, and automated blood pressure devices became standard in the latter half of the century. These innovations, combined with pharmacologic advances, markedly reduced anesthesia-related mortality, which fell from rates as high as 1 in 10,000 anesthetics in the 1940s to fewer than 1 in 100,000 today.

1.5.4 World Wars and Critical Care

The World Wars further accelerated anesthesiology's development. Anesthesiologists refined resuscitation techniques, pain management, and transfusion practices, many of which directly influenced the growth of intensive care medicine. The 1950s and 1960s saw the establishment of anesthesia as a recognized specialty in most Western countries, with the establishment of formal residency programs and professional societies.

1.6 The History of Anesthesia in the United States

1.6.1 Early Leadership

Following Morton's ether demonstration in Boston, the United States became a center of anesthetic innovation. Ether and chloroform were rapidly incorporated into American surgical practice, and hospitals across the country established anesthesia services. However, these were often ad hoc arrangements, with delivery by non-specialists.

1.6.2 Professionalization

The early twentieth century brought increasing recognition of anesthesia as a medical discipline. Ralph Waters, often regarded as the "father of academic anesthesiology" in the United States, established the first anesthesiology residency at the University of Wisconsin in 1927. He emphasized systematic training, research, and perioperative medicine, helping define anesthesiology as a specialty requiring medical judgment, not just technical skill.

1.6.3 Organizational Growth

The American Society of Anesthesiologists (ASA), founded as the Long Island Society of Anesthetists in 1905, grew into a national organization advocating for standards, education, and patient safety. In 1938, the American Board of Anesthesiology (ABA) was established, becoming one of the earliest specialty boards in the United States. These bodies formalized training requirements, certification, and research, cementing anesthesiology as a core medical specialty.

1.6.4 Workforce Structure

The United States also pioneered team-based models of care, integrating Certified Registered Nurse Anesthetists and later Anesthesiologist Assistants. This model remains distinctive, balancing physician leadership with advanced practice providers to expand access to anesthesia services nationwide.

1.7 Global Perspectives

While the United States played a central role in anesthesia's professionalization, advances were mirrored worldwide. European countries contributed innovations in pharmacology, monitoring, and pain medicine. In resource-limited settings, nurse anesthetists became the backbone of surgical anesthesia. Today, global initiatives focus on expanding safe anesthesia access, recognizing that millions of patients worldwide still lack reliable anesthetic care.

1.8 Modern Era: Beyond the Operating Room

In the contemporary era, anesthesiology extends far beyond intraoperative care. In the United States and globally, anesthesiologists lead in:

- *Critical care medicine*: Directing ICUs and advancing resuscitation science.
- *Pain medicine*: Chronic and cancer pain management.
- *Perioperative medicine*: Risk stratification, enhanced recovery programs, and multidisciplinary optimization.
- *Patient safety*: Leading simulation, quality improvement, and crisis resource management.
- *Advanced imaging*: Proficiency in transesophageal echocardiography and point-of-care ultrasound.

This expanded role highlights why internists benefit from understanding anesthesia's scope. Anesthesiologists are no longer confined to "putting patients to sleep" but rather function as perioperative physicians, intensivists, and patient safety leaders.

1.9 Conclusion

The history of anesthesia is not simply a narrative of pharmacologic discovery but a story of medicine's evolution toward safer, more humane, and more sophisticated care. From ether in 1846 to the integrated perioperative services of today, anesthesiology has continuously shaped the practice of modern medicine. For internists, appreciating this history provides context for collaboration, reinforces the importance of interprofessional communication, and deepens understanding of anesthesiology's role in patient care.

Key Takeaways

1. The discovery of ether anesthesia in 1846 revolutionized surgery and is regarded as the birth of modern anesthesia.
2. The introduction of intravenous agents and neuromuscular blockers transformed anesthesiology into a scientific discipline with precise physiological control.
3. Advances in monitoring (pulse oximetry and capnography) markedly reduced anesthesia-related mortality throughout the twentieth century.
4. In the United States, figures such as Ralph Waters, the ASA, and the ABA formalized anesthesiology as a specialty and expanded its scope.
5. Modern anesthesiology extends beyond the operating room, encompassing perioperative medicine, critical care, and patient safety leadership.

Suggested Reading

1. Wiklund RA, Rosenbaum SH. Anesthesiology. First of two parts. N Engl J Med. 1997;337(16):1132–41.
2. Wiklund RA, Rosenbaum SH. Anesthesiology. Second of two parts. N Engl J Med. 1997;337(17):1215–9.
3. Abhyankar RS, Jessop KM. From craft to profession: the development of modern anesthesiology. Mo Med. 2022;119(1):14–20.
4. Gawande A. Two hundred years of surgery. N Engl J Med. 2012;366(18):1716–23.
5. Robinson DH, Toledo AH. Historical development of modern anesthesia. J Invest Surg. 2012;25(3):141–9.
6. Borghi L. The monuments men: in the history of anesthesia, too. Anesthesiology. 2015;122(3):521–3.
7. Gaba DM. Anaesthesiology as a model for patient safety in health care. BMJ. 2000;320(7237):785–8.

The Anesthesia Workforce

2

2.1 Introduction

The delivery of safe anesthesia is a complex, highly technical, and knowledge-driven endeavor. It requires mastery of physiology, pharmacology, resuscitation science, advanced imaging, and crisis management. While anesthesia services can be provided by different categories of practitioners, anesthesiologists are physicians who complete rigorous medical school training, residency, and often an optional fellowship specialization. Anesthesiologists remain the only professionals trained to integrate the full spectrum of perioperative medicine, critical care, and pain management.

Understanding the composition of the anesthesia workforce is essential for internists. Internists frequently collaborate with anesthesia teams during preoperative evaluations, perioperative consultations, and in critical care environments. This chapter outlines the roles of anesthesiologists, certified registered nurse anesthetists (CRNAs), and anesthesiologist assistants (AAs), while also discussing the structure of team-based models of care.

2.2 Anesthesiologists as Perioperative Leaders

2.2.1 Training and Expertise

Anesthesiologists are physicians who undergo a minimum of:

- Four years of medical school, where they acquire a broad foundation in anatomy, physiology, pathology, and pharmacology
- Four years of residency training in anesthesiology, which includes rotations in anesthesia and its subspecialties (e.g., cardiac, pediatric, neuro, and obstetric), intensive care, and perioperative medicine

A. Mirrakhimov, *Anesthesiology Demystified for the Internist*,
https://doi.org/10.1007/978-3-032-16811-5_2

- Optional subspecialty fellowships (typically 1 year in duration) in adult cardiac anesthesiology, pediatric anesthesiology, pain medicine, critical care medicine, obstetric anesthesiology, or research

This pathway equips anesthesiologists to manage the entire perioperative continuum:

- *Preoperative*: risk stratification, optimization of comorbidities, coordination with internists, surgeons, and proceduralists
- *Intraoperative*: management of anesthesia depth, airway, hemodynamics, ventilation, transfusion, and crises
- *Postoperative*: postoperative care and intensive care unit management, pain control, recognition of complications, and their management

2.2.2 Breadth of Scope

Unlike other providers, anesthesiologists are uniquely qualified to:

- Manage patients with complex comorbidities (e.g., pulmonary hypertension, cardiomyopathy, and liver failure)
- Direct cardiac anesthesia and transesophageal echocardiography (TEE)
- Lead critical care units
- Provide acute and chronic pain management
- Innovate in patient safety science, simulation, and perioperative systems design

2.2.3 Leadership Role

The American Society of Anesthesiologists emphasizes the anesthesiologist's role as the perioperative physician. This role extends well and far beyond "putting patients to sleep." It involves guiding perioperative decision-making, anticipating complications, and ensuring patient safety across surgical and non-surgical settings.

Internists benefit from understanding that, although CRNAs and AAs can deliver anesthesia within certain frameworks, anesthesiologists remain the only professionals capable of independently managing the full complexity of perioperative care, especially in high-acuity and crisis situations.

2.3 Certified Registered Nurse Anesthetists

2.3.1 Training and Certification

CRNAs are advanced practice nurses who complete:

- A bachelor's degree in nursing
- At least 1 year of critical care nursing experience
- A graduate-level nurse anesthesia program (typically 3 years)
- National certification via the National Board of Certification and Recertification for Nurse Anesthetists

While CRNAs develop strong technical skills in anesthetic delivery, their training is fundamentally nursing-based, without the breadth of medical education, diagnostic reasoning, or systems-level expertise inherent to physician training.

2.3.2 Practice Environment

CRNAs provide anesthesia in a variety of settings, often in community hospitals, ambulatory centers, or rural facilities. In some states, governors have opted out of federal requirements for physician supervision, allowing CRNAs to practice independently. However, a large body of literature underscores the value of physician involvement, particularly in complex cases, emergencies, or high-acuity settings.

2.3.3 Scope Limitations

Although CRNAs provide valuable anesthesia care, they lack:

- Training in perioperative medical optimization
- Expertise in advanced imaging (e.g., TEE and POCUS)
- Comprehensive exposure to the management of rare but life-threatening complications (e.g., malignant hyperthermia, massive hemorrhage, and cardiac arrest under anesthesia)

Thus, while CRNAs are an important part of the workforce, their scope does not replace the breadth of anesthesiology as a medical specialty.

2.4 Anesthesiologist Assistants

2.4.1 Training and Certification

AAs are non-physician anesthesia providers educated in programs modeled after physician assistant curricula, but specific to anesthesia. Their pathway includes:

- A bachelor's degree with premedical coursework
- A 24–28-month master's program in anesthesia
- Certification through the National Commission for Certification of Anesthesiologist Assistants

2.4.2 Practice Environment

AAs work exclusively under the medical direction of anesthesiologists. Their role is designed to expand access to anesthesia care while ensuring physician oversight. They are not permitted to practice independently.

2.4.3 Scope of Practice

AAs can:

- Perform preoperative assessments under supervision
- Induce and maintain anesthesia under the direction of an anesthesiologist
- Assist with invasive monitoring, airway management, and postoperative care

Unlike CRNAs, AAs do not have an independent practice lobby. Their role is inherently tied to physician-led models of care.

2.5 Team-Based Models of Care

2.5.1 The Anesthesia Care Team Model

The Anesthesia Care Team (ACT) model is the most common workforce design in the United States. It integrates anesthesiologists, CRNAs, and AAs, with anesthesiologists providing medical direction and supervision. This model allows flexibility while preserving physician oversight for complex decision-making.

The benefits of the ACT model include the following:

- *Scalability*: Expands access to anesthesia care across different practice environments.

- *Safety*: Maintains physician involvement in diagnosis, planning, and crisis management.
- *Collaboration*: Leverages the technical expertise of CRNAs and AAs alongside physician leadership.

2.5.2 Independent Practice Debate

Some CRNA organizations advocate independent practice, arguing that it expands access in underserved areas. However, studies suggest that outcomes are best in physician-led or medically directed models, particularly in high-risk surgeries and patient populations with multiple comorbidities.

Internists should recognize that while CRNAs provide competent care in routine settings, the physician anesthesiologist's knowledge and ability to synthesize complex medical information remain indispensable.

2.6 Global Workforce Perspectives

Worldwide, anesthesia workforce structures vary:

- *High-income countries*: Predominantly physician anesthesiologists, often with nurse anesthetists in team-based roles.
- *Low- and middle-income countries (LMICs)*: Nurse anesthetists and non-physician providers often deliver the majority of anesthesia, with limited physician oversight. This reflects workforce shortages more than optimal design.

2.7 Conclusion

The anesthesia workforce is diverse, reflecting historical evolution, healthcare economics, and patient needs. CRNAs and AAs contribute meaningfully to anesthesia delivery, particularly in extending access. However, anesthesiologists remain the true perioperative leaders, with unparalleled training and expertise that spans preoperative evaluation, intraoperative management, critical care, and postoperative recovery.

For internists, understanding this structure clarifies why collaboration with anesthesiologists is essential. While team-based models ensure coverage, the physician anesthesiologist's presence guarantees the highest level of safety and the integration of complex medical decision-making.

In short, anesthesia is not simply the administration of drugs—it is the orchestration of physiology, pharmacology, and patient safety in real time. And in that orchestra, anesthesiologists remain the conductors.

Key Takeaways

1. Anesthesiologists are perioperative leaders, uniquely trained to manage complex physiology, crises, and multidisciplinary care.
2. CRNAs provide valuable anesthesia delivery, particularly in community and rural settings, but their scope is narrower than physician anesthesiologists.
3. AAs practice exclusively under the supervision of an anesthesiologist, extending access without independent practice.
4. The ACT model is the dominant U.S. structure, combining scalability and safety through physician-led oversight.
5. Global workforce structures differ, with physician shortages in LMICs leading to reliance on nurse anesthetists or non-physician providers.

Suggested Reading

1. Matsusaki T, Sakai T. The role of Certified Registered Nurse Anesthetists in the United States. J Anesth. 2011;25(5):734–40.
2. https://www.asahq.org/standards-and-practice-parameters/statement-on-the-anesthesia-care-team
3. Pinegar M, Townsend T. The role of anesthesiology assistants in the anesthesiology patient care team. Mo Med. 2019;116(1):63–6.
4. Gaba DM. Anaesthesiology as a model for patient safety in health care. BMJ. 2000;320(7237):785–8.

3 Anesthesiology and Its Subspecialties

3.1 Introduction

Anesthesiology is a broad specialty that extends well beyond "putting patients to sleep." Today, anesthesiologists are perioperative physicians, critical care experts, pain specialists, and leaders in safety and resuscitation science. The backbone of the anesthesiology workforce is the general anesthesiologist, who is trained to provide safe anesthesia for most adult and pediatric procedures. From that foundation, multiple subspecialties have developed to address the needs of complex patients and highly specialized surgeries.

For internists, appreciating the subspecialty structure of anesthesiology clarifies how anesthesia care is organized in different clinical contexts. Whether co-managing a patient with heart failure undergoing cardiac surgery, a pregnant patient with preeclampsia requiring cesarean delivery, or a liver transplant recipient with multiple comorbidities, internists inevitably interface with anesthesiologists and their subspecialty teams.

3.2 The Scope of General Anesthesiology

Board certification in general anesthesiology is awarded by the American Board of Anesthesiology (ABA) following completion of 4 years of anesthesiology residency training after medical school. Residency encompasses exposure to adult, pediatric, obstetric, neuro, trauma, regional, chronic pain, and cardiac anesthesia, as well as critical care rotations. Residents must also demonstrate competency in advanced airway management, invasive monitoring, mechanical ventilation, and perioperative medicine.

General anesthesiologists are qualified to:

- Provide anesthesia for most surgical cases (e.g., orthopedic, general, gynecologic, urologic, plastic, and ENT).

A. Mirrakhimov, *Anesthesiology Demystified for the Internist*,
https://doi.org/10.1007/978-3-032-16811-5_3

- Manage airways and provide mechanical ventilation.
- Deliver regional anesthesia (e.g., neuraxial and peripheral nerve blocks).
- Conduct preoperative evaluations and optimize patients' comorbidities.
- Manage acute perioperative complications.
- Provide anesthesia for non-operating room procedures such as endoscopy, interventional radiology, or cardiac catheterization.

Many general anesthesiologists practice in community hospitals, ambulatory surgery centers, and private practice groups. They frequently interface with internists for preoperative optimization of patients with chronic conditions such as heart failure, diabetes, or chronic obstructive pulmonary disease (COPD). While general anesthesiologists can manage most procedures, patients undergoing highly complex surgeries or those with unusual physiological demands are often cared for by fellowship-trained subspecialists.

3.3 Cardiac Anesthesiology

Cardiac anesthesiology is among the most highly specialized fields. They care for patients undergoing open heart surgery, structural heart interventions, thoracic aortic surgery, congenital cardiac surgery, and mechanical circulatory support procedures.

Internists, especially cardiologists and hospitalists, frequently collaborate with cardiac anesthesiologists in perioperative planning for patients with ischemic heart disease, cardiomyopathy, or valvular pathology. Understanding the cardiac anesthesiologist's role helps internists anticipate perioperative challenges and integrate chronic disease management with surgical planning.

3.3.1 Scope

- Management of anesthesia for coronary artery bypass grafting, valve replacements and repairs, aortic dissections, and congenital heart operations.
- Intraoperative use of transesophageal echocardiography (TEE) for diagnostic and surgical guidance.
- Care for patients on mechanical circulatory support, including extracorporeal membrane oxygenation, Impella, and durable left ventricular assist device.
- Expertise in perioperative management of patients with severe heart failure, pulmonary hypertension, and arrhythmias.

3.3.2 Board Certification and Practice

The ABA offers subspecialty certification in Adult Cardiac Anesthesiology, making it one of the formally recognized advanced areas within the field. In addition, cardiac anesthesiologists commonly pursue certification in Advanced Perioperative TEE through the National Board of Echocardiography. These specialists typically practice in tertiary academic medical centers or dedicated heart hospitals, where they provide anesthetic care for complex cardiac and thoracic procedures.

3.4 Critical Care Anesthesiology

Critical care medicine is a multidisciplinary field that has deep roots in anesthesiology. Many early intensive care units (ICUs) were established and directed by anesthesiologists, leveraging their expertise in airway management, mechanical ventilation, and resuscitation.

Internists frequently encounter anesthesiologist-intensivists in ICUs, especially when patients transition from surgical care to medical management. The shared language of physiology and hemodynamics strengthens collaboration between internists and anesthesiologist intensivists.

3.4.1 Scope

- Management of critically ill patients with shock, respiratory failure, and multi-organ dysfunction.
- Advanced ventilator strategies for acute respiratory distress syndrome (ARDS) and perioperative respiratory failure.
- Hemodynamic monitoring, vasoactive support, and resuscitation.
- Coordination of multidisciplinary care for sepsis, trauma, and perioperative critical illness.

3.4.2 Board Certification and Practice

The ABA offers board certification in Critical Care Medicine after a 1-year fellowship. Anesthesiology-trained intensivists practice in surgical, trauma, neurosurgical, cardiac, and mixed ICUs, often working alongside internists and pulmonologists.

3.5 Pediatric Anesthesiology

Pediatric anesthesia is a distinct and highly nuanced subspecialty, as children differ from adults in their physiology, pharmacology, and anatomy. These differences influence drug metabolism, airway management, and perioperative responses. Neonates and infants, in particular, require highly specialized expertise due to their unique developmental physiology and limited physiologic reserves.

3.5.1 Scope

- Anesthesia for neonates, infants, children, and adolescents.
- Perioperative management of congenital anomalies, pediatric airway disorders, and congenital heart disease.
- Pediatric regional anesthesia for postoperative pain.
- Perioperative care for children with complex syndromes or comorbidities.

3.5.2 Board Certification and Practice

The ABA offers board certification in Pediatric Anesthesiology following a 1-year fellowship. Pediatric anesthesiologists primarily practice in children's hospitals and large academic centers, where the surgical volumes justify subspecialty expertise.

3.6 Pain Medicine

Pain medicine is a multidisciplinary field that anesthesiologists helped establish and continue to lead. Unlike most anesthesia subspecialties, which are procedure- or setting-based, chronic pain medicine differs fundamentally in scope and practice. Rather than focusing on perioperative care, pain specialists manage patients longitudinally, often in outpatient clinics. Their work emphasizes diagnostic evaluation, multimodal pharmacotherapy, interventional procedures, and rehabilitation. This continuity of care and integration with primary and specialty medicine distinguishes pain medicine from the acute, episodic focus of general anesthesiology and most of its subspecialties.

Internists frequently serve as the first point of care for chronic pain patients. Anesthesiologist pain specialists provide advanced interventional and multimodal options, reducing reliance on long-term opioids and improving quality of life.

3.6.1 Scope

- Chronic non-cancer pain management (back pain, neuropathic pain, and complex regional pain syndrome).
- Cancer-related pain and palliative interventions.
- Interventional techniques: epidural steroid injections, nerve ablations, spinal cord stimulation, and intrathecal drug delivery systems.
- Multimodal pharmacologic strategies and opioid stewardship.

3.6.2 Board Certification and Practice

The ABA offers subspecialty certification in Pain Medicine, often after a 1-year fellowship (jointly accredited with other boards, such as Physical Medicine and Rehabilitation and Neurology). Pain physicians work in multidisciplinary pain clinics, academic centers, and community practices, often co-managing patients with internists and primary care physicians.

3.7 Obstetric Anesthesiology

Pregnancy introduces a range of unique physiological changes that affect nearly every organ system and have important anesthetic implications. Obstetric anesthesiologists play a critical role in ensuring the safety and well-being of both the mother and fetus during labor, delivery, cesarean section, and the peripartum period.

Internists often manage pregnant patients with chronic diseases (hypertension, diabetes, and congenital heart disease). Collaboration with obstetric anesthesiologists ensures safe anesthetic planning and peripartum management.

3.7.1 Scope

- Neuraxial analgesia for labor (epidural, spinal, and combined spinal–epidural).
- Cesarean delivery anesthesia, typically neuraxial but occasionally general.
- Management of high-risk pregnancies with preeclampsia, cardiomyopathy, or coagulopathies.
- Crisis response for maternal cardiac arrest, amniotic fluid embolism, and obstetric hemorrhage.

3.7.2 Board Certification and Practice

Unlike cardiac, pediatric, or pain anesthesiology, obstetric anesthesiology does not currently have ABA subspecialty certification. Fellowships are available but are not universally Accreditation Council for Graduate Medical Education (ACGME)-accredited. Obstetric anesthesiologists typically work in academic centers and tertiary care hospitals with high delivery volumes and complex obstetric populations.

3.8 Regional Anesthesiology and Acute Pain

Regional anesthesia provides targeted analgesia, minimizing systemic opioid requirements and promoting faster recovery. It encompasses not only perioperative pain management but also procedural, surgical, and trauma-related pain. Peripheral nerve blocks and neuraxial techniques are invaluable for orthopedic and abdominal surgery and play a key role in managing acute pain from rib fractures, limb injuries, and other traumatic conditions.

While many general anesthesiologists can safely and effectively perform standard regional blocks, anesthesiologists with advanced training in regional anesthesiology bring an additional level of reliability and precision. Their expertise allows for the selection and tailoring of more complex regional techniques, including ultrasound-guided and continuous catheter-based approaches, to optimize pain control and minimize complications.

For internists co-managing postoperative patients, regional anesthesia offers important downstream benefits—reducing respiratory depression, delirium, and thromboembolic complications associated with systemic opioid therapy. By providing focused, opioid-sparing analgesia, regional techniques enhance patient comfort, pulmonary function, and early mobilization across both surgical and nonsurgical settings.

3.8.1 Scope

- Ultrasound-guided peripheral nerve blocks (e.g., brachial plexus, femoral, and sciatic).
- Continuous catheter techniques for extended postoperative analgesia.
- Acute pain consultative services and enhanced recovery pathways.

3.8.2 Board Certification and Practice

Regional anesthesiology does not currently have ABA subspecialty certification, although fellowship training opportunities exist, many of which are non-ACGME-accredited. Regional anesthesiologists typically practice in academic institutions and high-volume surgical centers, where advanced regional programs support multimodal analgesia strategies and facilitate efficient, patient-centered anesthetic care.

3.9 Neuroanesthesiology

Neuroanesthesiology supports patients undergoing neurosurgery and interventional neuroradiology procedures. Many academic medical centers offer 1-year fellowship training programs in Neuroanesthesiology, providing advanced expertise in the anesthetic management of patients undergoing neurosurgical, spine, and interventional neuroradiologic procedures.

3.9.1 Scope

- Craniotomies for tumors, aneurysms, arteriovenous malformations, epilepsy, and traumatic brain injury.
- Management of intracranial pressure, cerebral perfusion, and neurophysiologic monitoring.
- Anesthesia for interventional procedures such as stroke thrombectomy.

3.9.2 Board Certification and Practice

There is no ABA subspecialty certification for Neuroanesthesiology. Fellowship programs exist, but many are not ACGME-accredited. Neuroanesthesiologists usually practice in academic centers and tertiary referral hospitals where neurosurgical volumes are high.

3.10 Trauma Anesthesiology

Trauma anesthesiology is a high-intensity field at the intersection of resuscitation and surgical anesthesia. A limited number of major academic trauma centers offer 1-year fellowship programs in Trauma Anesthesiology, providing advanced training in the perioperative and critical care management of patients with severe traumatic injuries.

3.10.1 Scope

- Rapid airway and anesthetic management for multiply injured patients.
- Massive transfusion protocols and hemostatic resuscitation.
- Intraoperative management of unstable trauma patients.
- Use of TEE and point of care ultrasound (POCUS) to guide real-time resuscitation.

3.10.2 Board Certification and Practice

There is no ABA subspecialty certification in Trauma Anesthesiology. Fellowships exist, often non-ACGME-accredited. Trauma anesthesiologists typically practice in Level I trauma centers and in military medicine.

3.11 Transplant Anesthesiology

Transplant anesthesiology requires mastery of complex physiology and perioperative management of end-stage organ failure. Several major academic medical centers offer 1-year fellowship training in Transplant Anesthesiology, focusing primarily on the perioperative management of patients undergoing abdominal organ transplantation, including liver, kidney, and multivisceral transplants. Thoracic organ transplantation—such as heart and lung transplantation—is typically managed by cardiac anesthesiologists, given the specialized expertise required in cardiopulmonary physiology and mechanical circulatory support.

Internists, particularly nephrologists, hepatologists, and endocrinologists, often coordinate long-term care for transplant patients. Collaboration with transplant anesthesiologists ensures perioperative safety during these highly complex procedures.

3.11.1 Scope

- Anesthesia for liver, kidney, and pancreas transplantation.
- Perioperative management of massive transfusion, coagulopathy, and multi-organ failure.
- Integration with transplant medicine teams regarding immunosuppression and long-term care.

3.11.2 Board Certification and Practice

There is no ABA subspecialty certification in Transplant Anesthesiology. Fellowships are available but typically non-ACGME-accredited. Transplant anesthesiologists work in large academic centers and transplant-designated hospitals.

3.12 Conclusion

The breadth of anesthesiology is extraordinary. General anesthesiologists provide safe anesthesia for most surgical patients, but subspecialists extend the specialty's reach into some of the most demanding areas of modern medicine—cardiac surgery, intensive care, pediatrics, chronic pain, obstetrics, neurosurgery, trauma, and transplantation.

Board certification exists for General Anesthesiology, Adult Cardiac Anesthesiology, Pediatric Anesthesiology, Pain Medicine, and Critical Care Medicine, but other important subspecialties, such as obstetric, neuro, regional, trauma, and transplant anesthesiology, are currently not formally recognized by the

ABA, despite their widespread training programs. Many of these fellowships are non-ACGME-accredited, reflecting variability in recognition across subspecialties.

Subspecialists typically practice in academic centers, tertiary hospitals, and specialized care units, while general anesthesiologists often form the backbone of anesthesia delivery in community hospitals and ambulatory settings.

For internists, recognizing the scope and structure of anesthesiology's subspecialties facilitates better collaboration. Whether preparing a patient for cardiac surgery, co-managing sepsis in the ICU, or caring for a patient after a liver transplant, internists and anesthesiologists share responsibility for optimizing outcomes.

Ultimately, anesthesiology's subspecialties highlight a central truth: anesthesiologists are not merely providers of anesthesia, but comprehensive perioperative physicians whose expertise spans the operating room, ICU, pain clinic, and beyond.

Key Takeaways

1. General anesthesiologists provide most of the perioperative care, but subspecialists address high-acuity and complex surgical populations.
2. Board-recognized subspecialties include adult cardiac anesthesiology, pediatric anesthesiology, pain medicine, and critical care medicine.
3. Non-board-certified subspecialties such as obstetric, regional, neuro, trauma, and transplant anesthesiology remain essential through fellowship training.
4. Collaboration between internists and anesthesiology subspecialists is vital in managing patients with complex comorbidities, critical illness, and specialized surgical needs.
5. Anesthesiology's scope extends beyond the OR, encompassing ICU management, pain medicine, and systems-level leadership in patient safety.

Suggested Reading

1. https://www.theaba.org/
2. https://careersinmedicine.aamc.org/explore-options/specialty-profiles/anesthesiology
3. Desjardins G, Cahalan MK. Subspecialty accreditation: is being special good? Curr Opin Anaesthesiol. 2007;20(6):572–5.
4. Rockoff MA, Hall SC. Subspecialty training in pediatric anesthesiology: what does it mean? Anesth Analg. 1997;85(6):1185–90.
5. Hochberg U, Sharon H, Bahir I, et al. Pain management—a decade's perspective of a new subspecialty. J Pain Res. 2021;14:923–30.
6. Tsai A, Faloye A, Bodmer N, et al. Preparing for the adult cardiac anesthesiology subspecialty certification: recognition of expertise in cardiac anesthesiology. J Cardiothorac Vasc Anesth. 2023;37(12):2405–8.
7. Flynn BC, Hicks MH, Jabaley CS, et al. Sustainability of the subspecialty of anesthesiology critical care: an expert consensus and review of the literature. J Cardiothorac Vasc Anesth. 2024;38(8):1753–9.
8. To L, Ye M, Chang S, et al. The evolution of teaching and learning regional anesthesia at every career stage: the U.S. perspective. Saudi J Anaesth. 2025;19(2):174–80.

9. Zhitny VP, Do K, Kawana E, et al. Assessment and recommendations for website platforms of neuroanesthesiology fellowship programs. J Neurosurg Anesthesiol. 2024;36(4):341–5.
10. Kuczkowski KM. A review of obstetric anesthesia in the new millennium: where we are and where is it heading? Curr Opin Obstet Gynecol. 2010;22(6):482–6.
11. https://www.asahq.org/about-asa/governance-and-committees/asa-committees/committee-on-trauma-and-emergency-preparedness-cotep/trauma-anesthesiology
12. Sharma S, Saner FH, Bezinover D. A brief history of liver transplantation and transplant anesthesia. BMC Anesthesiol. 2022;22:363.

Introduction: Why Internists Need to Understand the Basics of Anesthesia Practice

4

4.1 The Expanding Role of Internists in Perioperative Care

- *Demographics*: Surgical patients are older, frailer, and carry a higher burden of chronic medical diseases. Internists, especially hospitalists, are increasingly tasked with perioperative evaluation and co-management.
- *Knowledge gap*: Surveys show that internists often lack confidence in interpreting anesthetic risks, medication interactions, or anesthesia reports (e.g., transesophageal echocardiography (TEE) and echocardiography).
- *Collaborative model*: Perioperative medicine is evolving as a shared domain of anesthesiologists, internists, and surgeons, emphasizing communication and continuity.

4.2 The Importance of Basic Anesthesia Knowledge for Internists

4.2.1 Preoperative Assessment

Internists often serve as the first physicians to evaluate surgical risk. While perioperative guidelines exist (e.g., American College of Cardiology (ACC)/American Heart Association (AHA) and American Society ofAnesthesiologists (ASA)), anesthetic considerations, patient-specific nuances of airway anatomy, anticipated hemodynamic shifts, and implications of neuraxial blockade are often overlooked unless internists have basic anesthesia knowledge.

4.2.2 Medication Management

Perioperative continuation or withdrawal of beta-blockers, angiotensin converting enzyme (ACE) inhibitors, anticoagulants, and psychotropics can dramatically

A. Mirrakhimov, *Anesthesiology Demystified for the Internist*,
https://doi.org/10.1007/978-3-032-16811-5_4

influence anesthetic course. Internists' prescribing decisions directly impact perioperative anesthetic care.

4.2.3 Risk Stratification

Cardiac, pulmonary, and renal risk indices intersect with anesthesia management. An internist who understands how anesthesia alters physiology (e.g., positive-pressure ventilation and sympathetic blockade) provides more nuanced risk estimates.

4.2.4 Intraoperative Awareness

While internists are not in the operating room, understanding common monitoring modalities (e.g., invasive arterial lines, central venous catheters, and intraoperative TEE) enables better interpretation of anesthetic records and postoperative anesthesiology notes.

4.2.5 Postoperative Co-management

Complications such as delirium, hypoxemia, myocardial infarction, and acute kidney injury typically require an internist's input. Knowledge of how anesthetics contribute to these complications informs better diagnostic and therapeutic strategies.

4.3 Airway, Acute Physiology, and Drug Effects: The Missing Link for Internists

- *Airway*: Internists frequently encounter notes such as "difficult airway," but many do not appreciate its implications and importance for perioperative care.
- *Cardiovascular physiology*: Induction agents, volatile anesthetics, and opioids can all contribute to hypotension through multiple mechanisms, including depression of myocardial contractility and alterations in vascular tone. Recognizing these pharmacologic effects is essential for understanding and managing perioperative hemodynamic instability.
- *Neuraxial techniques*: Understanding sympathectomy and perioperative fluid shifts is essential for internists involved in managing postoperative hypotension, as these factors often underlie hemodynamic instability following anesthesia and surgery.
- *Drug interactions*: Chronically administered medications—such as selective serotonin reuptake inhibitors, monoamine oxidase inhibitors, clonidine, amiodarone, and numerous others—can have significant pharmacologic interactions that may potentiate or adversely interact with anesthetic agents, resulting in potentially serious perioperative complications.

4.4 The Multidisciplinary Imperative

Perioperative medicine is strongest when internists and anesthesiologists collaborate.

- *Shared language*: Familiarity with common anesthetic terminology—such as monitored anesthesia care, bispectral index (an adjunct monitor of anesthetic depth), and ASA physical status classification—enhances interdisciplinary communication and facilitates more effective collaboration in perioperative care.
- *Continuity of care*: Internists ensure long-term medical optimization (e.g., diabetes, heart failure, anticoagulation, etc.), while anesthesiologists manage acute intraoperative physiology.
- *Safety*: Cross-disciplinary understanding reduces errors and enhances perioperative outcomes.

4.5 Goals of This Text

1. Provide internists with a structured overview of anesthetic principles relevant to perioperative care
2. Highlight decision points where internist input is critical, such as medication management, comorbidity optimization, and postoperative complication management
3. Bridge knowledge gaps between anesthesiology and internal medicine by using clear language, case vignettes, and practical algorithms
4. Support collaborative practice models, empowering internists to engage in informed discussions with anesthesiologists and surgeons

Key Takeaways

- Internists are increasingly central to perioperative care due to aging and surgical patients with complex comorbid conditions.
- Limited exposure to anesthesiology in internal medicine training creates knowledge gaps that can affect perioperative safety.
- Understanding basic anesthesia principles (e.g., airway, physiology, drug effects, and monitoring) equips internists to provide better preoperative evaluation and postoperative co-management.
- Collaboration between internists and anesthesiologists requires a shared vocabulary and mutual understanding.

Suggested Reading

1. Wijeysundera DN, Pearse RM, Shulman MA, et al. Assessment of functional capacity before major non-cardiac surgery: an international, prospective cohort study. Lancet. 2018;391(10140):2631–40.
2. Leibowitz AB, Silverstein JH. Anesthesia: what the internist needs to know. Mt Sinai J Med. 1991;58(1):9–15.
3. Potyk DK, Raudaskoski P. Overview of anesthesia for primary care physicians. West J Med. 1998;168(6):517–21.

Part II

The Perioperative Environment

Dynamics of the Operating and Procedure Room

5

5.1 Introduction

The operating room (OR) and procedural suites are unique microenvironments in healthcare, highly structured, technologically complex, and utterly dependent on team performance. Decisions must be made rapidly, communication must be precise, and safety must be prioritized above all else. Unlike most clinical settings, OR care is delivered by multiple professionals, surgeons, and surgical trainees (e.g., residents and fellows), anesthesiologists (including residents and fellows), certified registered nurse anesthetists (CRNAs) or anesthesiologist assistants (AAs), nurses, technologists, and support staff—working in synchrony under conditions of significant physiologic and procedural risk.

For internists, who often engage with patients before or after surgery, understanding the dynamics of the OR is important. Internists are frequently asked to optimize patients preoperatively and to manage postoperative complications in the intensive care unit (ICU) or ward. Appreciating the collaborative structure of the OR helps contextualize perioperative decisions, anticipate sources of complication, and enable high-value communication with perioperative teams.

This chapter reviews the roles and interactions of surgical and procedural teams, the critical contributions of circulating and scrub nurses, and, centrally, the integration of the anesthesia team, including attending anesthesiologists, trainees (residents and fellows), CRNAs, and AAs.

A. Mirrakhimov, *Anesthesiology Demystified for the Internist*,
https://doi.org/10.1007/978-3-032-16811-5_5

5.2 Surgical and Procedural Teams

5.2.1 Composition

At the core of the OR is the surgical team, which typically includes:

- *Attending surgeon*—responsible for the operative plan, execution, and outcomes
- *Surgical trainees* (residents, fellows)—perform portions of the operation under supervision and manage perioperative tasks
- *Advanced practice providers* (surgical physician assistants (PAs)/nurse practitioners (NPs))—assist with preparation, intraoperative tasks, and postoperative care
- *Specialized support staff* (e.g., perfusionists for cardiac cases, radiology technicians in hybrid ORs, and device representatives for implants)

5.2.2 Workflow

Coordination begins in the preoperative area, where surgeons, anesthesiologists, and nursing teams align on patient-specific risks, equipment needs, and intraoperative milestones. During the procedure, surgeons communicate critical points—anticipated blood loss, clamping, reperfusion, insufflation, cementing, or positioning changes—so the anesthesia and nursing teams can anticipate physiologic consequences and resource needs.

5.2.3 Communication and Safety

The World Health Organization (WHO) Surgical Safety Checklist establishes structured communication at sign-in, time-out, and sign-out. These checkpoints foster a shared mental model of the patient, procedure, and potential hazards. Standardized briefings reduce ambiguity, facilitate anticipation of crises, and are associated with improved patient outcomes.

5.3 Circulating and Scrub Nurses

5.3.1 Circulating Nurses

The circulating nurse orchestrates flow, safety, and logistics:

- Verifies identity, consent, and site/side.
- Ensures sterility and environmental safety.
- Procures equipment, blood products, and medications.
- Documents intraoperative events and communications.
- Serves as the liaison between the sterile field and external resources (e.g., blood bank).

Circulators also maintain situational awareness and a calm, structured environment during crises, advocating for the anesthetized patient who cannot speak for themselves.

5.3.2 Scrub Nurses and Surgical Technologists

Scrub team members are part of the sterile field. They prepare instruments, anticipate steps, and maintain sterile technique. Their vigilance prevents contamination and keeps the operation efficient. In bleeding or time-critical situations, scrub accuracy and speed are directly linked to outcomes.

5.3.3 Team Dynamics

The collaboration between scrub, circulating, and anesthesia teams is often underappreciated outside the OR. In hemorrhage, for example, scrub personnel deliver the correct instruments swiftly; circulating nurses mobilize blood, equipment, and additional personnel; and anesthesia teams activate massive transfusion, secure lines, and stabilize hemodynamics. That synchronized choreography can be decisive for survival.

5.4 Anesthesia Team Integration

5.4.1 Composition and Roles

The "anesthesia team" encompasses:

- *Attending anesthesiologists* (physician perioperative leaders)
- *Anesthesiology residents* (physician trainees with graduated responsibility)
- *Anesthesiology fellows* (subspecialty physicians in advanced training—for example, cardiac, pediatric, critical care, obstetric, regional, neuro, and pain)
- *CRNAs* and *AAs* (non-physician anesthesia professionals practicing independently or under medical direction, depending on the model and jurisdiction)

Regardless of configuration, the attending anesthesiologist bears responsibility for medical leadership, complex decision-making, and crisis management.

5.4.2 Core Responsibilities of the Anesthesia Service

- *Airway and ventilation*: securing the airway, managing oxygenation/ventilation, lung-protective strategies when indicated
- *Hemodynamics*: titration of anesthetics, fluids, vasoactive drugs, and blood products; invasive monitoring; prevention/management of instability

- *Analgesia and hypnosis*: aligning anesthetic depth and analgesia with surgical stimuli; balancing multimodal regimens
- *Monitoring*: continuous interpretation of ECG, blood pressure, SpO_2, capnography, temperature, neuromuscular function; advanced monitors as needed
- *Crisis response*: leadership in malignant hyperthermia, anaphylaxis, local anesthetic systemic toxicity, hemorrhage, embolism, or cardiac arrest
- *Emergence and recovery*: safe wake-up, timely extubation when appropriate, handoff to post operative care unit (PACU)/intensive care unit (ICU) with clear plans and contingencies
- *Advocacy*: representing the patient's physiologic interests while the surgeon focuses on the field

5.4.3 Anesthesiology Residents: Roles, Supervision, and Safety

Residents are physicians in training who participate in:

- Preoperative evaluation (history/physical, risk stratification, medication reconciliation, optimization plans)
- Induction, maintenance, and emergence under supervision, including line placement, advanced airway techniques, and regional anesthesia
- Real-time data interpretation and crisis management with faculty guidance
- Structured handoffs to PACU/ICU and postoperative follow-up

Residents function under graduated responsibility: supervision intensity is tailored to case complexity and trainee competency. Critical portions (e.g., induction, emergence, and major hemodynamic transitions) are directly supervised; other phases may be indirectly supervised with immediate availability, in accordance with institutional policy and national standards. This model balances education and redundancy, increasing team bandwidth and resilience during high-acuity events. Simulation and debriefing reinforce non-technical skills—communication, resource management, and leadership—shown to impact outcomes in dynamic domains like the OR.

5.4.4 Anesthesiology Fellows: Advanced Expertise and Team Leadership

Fellows are board-eligible/board-certified anesthesiologists pursuing subspecialty training. They frequently:

- Lead advanced procedures (e.g., comprehensive TEE in cardiac cases; complex pediatric airways; advanced neurophysiologic monitoring; high-risk obstetric neuraxial techniques; and regional catheter programs)

- Supervise and teach residents, serving as a proximal resource while escalating to the attending for strategic decisions
- Coordinate subspecialty services (e.g., cardiac anesthesia line-ups, block teams, and ICU consults), smoothing flow and throughput

Fellows add depth and surge capacity during crises—an extra pair of expert hands and eyes—while elevating the team's capability to anticipate and mitigate risk.

5.4.5 CRNAs and AAs Within the Team

CRNAs and AAs provide high-value anesthesia care within the local practice model. In anesthesia care team arrangements, the attending anesthesiologist provides medical direction and supervision, ensuring consistent application of diagnostic judgment, crisis leadership, and systems integration across multiple rooms. Clear role delineation and bidirectional communication are essential to safety and efficiency.

5.4.6 Collaboration with Surgical and Nursing Teams

Integration is fundamental: surgeons rely on anesthesia for stable conditions during delicate steps, while anesthesia relies on surgeons to telegraph physiologic stressors. Circulating and scrub teams depend on anesthesia for precise cues about urgent needs (e.g., blood, vasopressors, warming devices, or specialized equipment). High-reliability communication—closed-loop verification, explicit contingency plans, and shared timing—underpins safe performance.

5.5 The Procedural Suite Beyond the OR

Modern anesthesia extends far beyond the operating theater, into:

- Endoscopy suites (EGD, colonoscopy, and ERCP)
- Interventional radiology (embolization, TIPS, and complex ablations)
- Cardiac catheterization and structural heart labs (TAVR, MitraClip, and EP ablations)
- Electroconvulsive therapy and radiation therapy suites

These non-operating room anesthesia (NORA) environments pose at least the same risks as the OR environment, such as airway compromise and hemodynamic instability, but may have less support systems in place due to remote location from the ORs (see Chap. 6 for more information). Anesthesiology residents and fellows rotate through NORA under faculty supervision, helping standardize safety practices (portable difficult-airway carts, capnography, and rescue pathways) while maintaining throughput. For internists frequently consulted in these areas, recognizing the anesthesia team's role clarifies risk discussions and discharge criteria.

5.6 Team Dynamics and Patient Safety

Decades of research link communication failures, not technical incompetence—to a large share of preventable harm in the OR. Teams mitigate this through:

- Pre-briefs, time-outs, and debriefs aligned with checklists (e.g., WHO)
- Crisis resource management (CRM) training to optimize leadership, situational awareness, and workload distribution
- Simulation for rare but catastrophic events (malignant hyperthermia, massive hemorrhage and operating room fire), which strengthens role clarity and muscle memory
- Standardized handoffs (e.g., PACU/ICU templates and closed-loop read-backs) that preserve critical information and intent

In academic centers, the presence of residents and fellows can enhance safety via redundancy (extra hands during instability), vigilance, and rapid mobilization of resources in the event of a crisis. Faculty oversight aligns training with safety, and structured debriefs convert cases into learning that propagates across the system.

5.7 Conclusion

The OR and procedural suites are among the most complex, high-reliability environments in medicine. Success depends on a cohesive, multidisciplinary team: surgeons directing the operative field; scrub and circulating nurses ensuring sterility, coordination, and logistics; and anesthesia teams safeguarding physiology, analgesia, and crisis response. Within anesthesia, attending anesthesiologists, residents, fellows, CRNAs, and AAs function as a coordinated unit—balancing medical leadership, education, and efficient flow.

For internists, understanding these dynamics is not merely academic. It illuminates the rationale behind preoperative optimization, explains intraoperative constraints and physiological perturbations, and clarifies postoperative trajectories. By recognizing how OR teams communicate, anticipate, and recover from stressors—and by appreciating the structured roles of anesthesia trainees alongside attendings—internists can contribute to safer handoffs, more targeted consultations, and better outcomes across the perioperative continuum.

Key Takeaways

1. The OR and procedural suites require tightly coordinated teamwork among surgeons, anesthesiologists, nurses, and technologists.
2. Circulating and scrub nurses play critical roles in maintaining sterility, logistics, and efficiency, especially during crises.
3. The anesthesia team leads physiologic management and crisis response, ensuring patient safety across the perioperative continuum.
4. Tools such as the WHO Surgical Safety Checklist and CRM training improve communication, reduce errors, and strengthen resilience.
5. For internists, understanding OR dynamics enhances collaboration, contextualizes perioperative decisions, and supports safer transitions of care.

Suggested Reading

1. Lingard L, Espin S, Whyte S, et al. Communication failures in the operating room: an observational classification of recurrent types and effects. Qual Saf Health Care. 2004;13(5):330–4.
2. Gaba DM. Anaesthesiology as a model for patient safety in health care. BMJ. 2000;320(7237):785–8.
3. Wahr JA, Prager RL, Abernathy JH, et al. Patient safety in the cardiac operating room: human factors and teamwork: a scientific statement from the American Heart Association. Circulation. 2013;128(10):1139–69.
4. Weiser TG, Haynes AB, Dziekan G, et al. Effect of a 19-item surgical safety checklist during urgent operations in a global patient population. Ann Surg. 2010;251(5):976–80.
5. Manser T. Teamwork and patient safety in dynamic domains of healthcare: a review of the literature. Acta Anaesthesiol Scand. 2009;53(2):143–51.

Non-Operating Room Anesthesia: Endoscopy, Catheterization Laboratory, Interventional Radiology, and Magnetic Resonance Imaging

6

6.1 Introduction

Over the past several decades, the demand for anesthesia services has expanded well beyond the confines of the traditional operating room (OR). Advances in technology, minimally invasive procedures, and patient preferences for less invasive alternatives have fueled a surge in diagnostic and therapeutic interventions performed outside the OR. Collectively, these practices are known as non-operating room anesthesia (NORA).

NORA encompasses anesthesia provided in endoscopy suites, cardiac catheterization and electrophysiology labs, interventional radiology (IR) suites, magnetic resonance imaging (MRI) and computed tomography (CT) scanners, and other procedural areas. These cases present unique challenges because they are performed in environments not specifically designed for anesthesia.

For internists, awareness of NORA is important. Many patients undergoing these procedures have significant comorbidities, and internists are often consulted for pre-procedural risk assessment or for managing complications post-procedure. Understanding the anesthesiologist's challenges in these settings helps internists appreciate peri-procedural risks and the value of collaborative care.

6.2 The Growth of NORA

- Several factors explain the rapid growth and increasing demand for NORA: *Shift toward minimally invasive procedures*: Endovascular stents, percutaneous valve replacements, and interventional oncology procedures increasingly replace open surgeries.
- *Expanded diagnostic imaging*: MRI and CT play central roles in evaluating neurological, oncological, and cardiovascular disease.
- *Outpatient demand*: Gastrointestinal endoscopy volumes have grown exponentially with widespread colon cancer screening and surveillance.

A. Mirrakhimov, *Anesthesiology Demystified for the Internist*,
https://doi.org/10.1007/978-3-032-16811-5_6

- *Aging population*: Older patients with multiple comorbidities are undergoing more complex procedures, often requiring anesthesia involvement for safety.

Currently, NORA accounts for over 50% of all anesthetics administered in the United States. Despite its prevalence, these environments often lack the infrastructure, personnel, and ergonomics of a traditional OR, creating unique risks.

6.3 Challenges of NORA

6.3.1 Remote and Isolated Locations

Unlike ORs, which are clustered and equipped for immediate emergency response, NORA suites are often located in separate hospital wings, basements, or outpatient facilities. This geographic isolation means:

- Delays in obtaining additional help during emergencies
- Longer response times for code teams or rapid transfusion services
- Limited availability of specialized airway carts or difficult airway devices unless specifically transported

6.3.2 Poor Ergonomics and Layout

NORA spaces are primarily designed for proceduralists and imaging equipment, not anesthesiologists. As a result:

- Limited space around the patient for anesthesia machines and monitoring equipment
- Restricted access to the airway—common in MRI gantries, prone interventional procedures, or fluoroscopy tables
- Radiation exposure in cath labs and IR requires additional protective gear, further hindering mobility

These constraints significantly complicate anesthetic management, particularly in crises requiring airway access or resuscitation.

6.3.3 Unfamiliar or Limited Support Staff

Unlike OR circulators and scrub nurses, procedural staff in NORA suites may have limited experience assisting anesthesiologists. Radiology or cardiology technicians may not be trained in tasks such as:

- Setting up suction or intravenous access

- Assisting with emergency airway management, including retrieving medications and bringing necessary equipment
- Assisting with patient positioning or transferring unstable patients

This lack of familiarity can slow emergency responses. It underscores the importance of pre-procedural briefings, role assignments, and simulation-based training for NORA teams.

6.3.4 Equipment and Monitoring Limitations

- Not all NORA sites are equipped with full American Society of Anesthesiologists (ASA)-standard monitors, though guidelines require them.
- MRI presents unique challenges—standard monitors, infusion pumps, and ventilators are unsafe within the magnetic field, requiring specialized MRI-compatible equipment.
- In some outpatient endoscopy centers, anesthesia workstations may be less sophisticated, with limited capacity for invasive monitoring or rapid transfusion.

6.3.5 Patient Factors

Patients referred for NORA procedures often have high comorbidity burdens. For example:

- Endoscopy patients may have advanced pulmonary disease, cirrhosis, or cardiac dysfunction.
- Cath lab patients frequently have severe coronary disease, arrhythmias, or cardiogenic shock.
- IR procedures often involve oncology patients with malnutrition, anemia, or coagulopathies.

These patients would often be classified as ASA III–IV (see Chap. 7 for more information), underscoring the need for anesthesiologists with advanced expertise rather than minimal sedation alone.

6.4 NORA in Specific Settings

6.4.1 Endoscopy Suites

Procedures: Colonoscopy, esophagogastroduodenoscopy (EGD), Endoscopic Retrograde Cholangiopancreatography (ERCP), endoscopic ultrasound.

Challenges:

- High throughput pressures (multiple cases per day).
- Risk of aspiration in patients with incomplete fasting, delayed gastric emptying, or upper gastrointestinal bleeding. Prolonged prone positioning in ERCP complicates airway access.
- Sedation and monitored anesthesia care are commonly utilized, but general anesthesia may be required for high-risk or complex cases.

6.4.2 Cardiac Catheterization and Electrophysiology Labs

Procedures: Coronary angiography, percutaneous coronary intervention (PCI), transcatheter aortic valve replacement (TAVR), MitraClip, and atrial fibrillation ablations.

Challenges:

- Patients often have severe structural heart disease or decompensated heart failure.
- Hemodynamic instability during balloon inflation (e.g., aspect of TAVR procedure), valve deployment, or ablation.
- Need for TEE in structural heart cases, requiring specialized anesthesia expertise.
- Radiation exposure necessitates shielding and awareness of occupational risks.

6.4.3 Interventional Radiology

Procedures: Embolization, Transjugular Intrahepatic Portosystemic Shunt (TIPS), tumor ablations, and trauma interventions.

Challenges:

- Many patients are coagulopathic or hemodynamically unstable.
- Positioning may be unconventional (prone, lateral, on angiography tables with limited access).
- Cases can be lengthy and unpredictable, requiring flexibility in anesthetic planning.
- Emergency IR cases may need to get started with limited preoperative evaluation.

6.4.4 MRI and Other Imaging Suites

Procedures: MRI for pediatrics, neurology, and oncology; interventional MRI-guided procedures.

Challenges:

- Airway access is severely limited once the patient is inside the scanner.
- Strict restrictions on ferromagnetic equipment.

- Noise and confined space complicate monitoring and vigilance.
- Pediatric MRI often requires general anesthesia or deep sedation, raising airway and emergence concerns.

6.5 Patient Safety in NORA

Despite its challenges, NORA can be delivered safely with careful planning and adherence to guidelines:

- ASA Standards for Basic Monitoring apply equally to NORA as to the OR.
- Pre-procedural checklists should verify equipment, suction, airway tools, and emergency drugs.
- Clear communication with proceduralists ensures early warning of physiologic stressors.
- Simulation and staff training improve crisis responses in remote sites.
- Appropriate triage is crucial patients with extreme comorbidities or instability may be safer in hybrid ORs rather than remote NORA locations.

6.6 Conclusion

NORA represents a rapidly expanding domain of anesthesiology, essential to modern procedural medicine. It is defined not by location but by challenges: remote sites, poor ergonomics, limited support staff, unfamiliar environments, and high-acuity patients. Anesthesiologists adapt to these challenges by applying the same safety standards and vigilance as in the OR, often under more difficult circumstances.

For internists, awareness of NORA's demands is critical. Patients undergoing endoscopy, cath lab, IR, or MRI procedures often have significant comorbidities and rely on close collaboration between internists and anesthesiologists. By understanding the unique environment and risks of NORA, internists can partner more effectively in perioperative care, ultimately improving patient safety and outcomes.

Key Takeaways

1. NORA now accounts for over 50% of all anesthetics administered in the United States, driven by the growth of minimally invasive procedures and advances in imaging technologies. Remote locations, poor ergonomics, and limited staff support distinguish NORA environments from the OR and increase risk during emergencies.
2. Patients undergoing NORA procedures often have high comorbidity burdens, requiring careful pre-procedural optimization.
3. ASA monitoring standards apply fully to NORA, with additional safeguards such as MRI-compatible equipment and structured checklists.
4. Collaboration between internists and anesthesiologists is critical for perioperative planning, complication management, and patient safety in NORA settings.

Suggested Reading

1. Metzner J, Posner KL, Domino KB. The risk and safety of anesthesia at remote locations: the US closed claims analysis. Curr Opin Anaesthesiol. 2009;22(4):502–8.
2. American Society of Anesthesiologists. Standards for basic anesthetic monitoring. ASA House of Delegates; 2020. https://www.asahq.org/standards-and-practice-parameters/standards-for-basic-anesthetic-monitoring.
3. Schroeck H, Welch TA, Rovner MS, et al. Anesthetic challenges and outcomes for procedures in the intraoperative magnetic resonance imaging suite: a systematic review. J Clin Anesth. 2019;54:89–101.
4. Primm A, Anca D. Updates in non-operating room anesthesia. Curr Opin Anaesthesiol. 2025;38(3):297–302.

7 Preoperative Assessment and Optimization: History, Risk Stratification, and Special Considerations

7.1 Introduction

Preoperative assessment and optimization are fundamental to safe perioperative medicine. For internists and anesthesiologists alike, preoperative evaluation serves three essential purposes: to identify and quantify perioperative risks, to optimize comorbid conditions where possible, and to facilitate shared decision-making regarding surgical appropriateness and periprocedural planning.

Recent guidelines, including the 2024 American Heart Association (AHA)/American College of Cardiology (ACC)/American College of Surgeons (ACS)/Society for Cardiovascular Anesthesiologists (SCA) perioperative cardiovascular evaluation document, emphasize a stepwise, individualized approach rather than universal testing. The contemporary paradigm balances the risk of surgical delay against the need for careful preoperative optimization.

7.2 History and Physical Examination

7.2.1 History

A thorough history remains the cornerstone of preoperative assessment. Key components include the following:

- *Functional status*: Measured in metabolic equivalents (METs). Patients able to perform >4 METs of activity (climbing one flight of stairs, walking up a hill) generally tolerate surgery better.
- *Comorbidities*: Cardiac disease, pulmonary disease, renal impairment, diabetes, and prior stroke strongly influence risk.
- *Medication history*: Including anticoagulants, antiplatelets, antihypertensives, and insulin, among many others.

A. Mirrakhimov, *Anesthesiology Demystified for the Internist*,
https://doi.org/10.1007/978-3-032-16811-5_7

- *Prior anesthetic history*: Previous airway complications and difficult intubation, postoperative nausea/vomiting, malignant hyperthermia, or pseudocholinesterase deficiency.
- *Social history*: Tobacco, alcohol, and recreational drug use, all of which affect perioperative physiology and recovery.

7.2.2 Physical Examination

The examination should focus on:

- *Airway assessment*: Mallampati score, neck mobility, mouth opening, dentition, and history of obstructive sleep apnea. This assessment is essential for identifying patients with a potentially difficult airway.
- *Cardiopulmonary system*: Baseline heart rate, blood pressure, lung auscultation, and signs of heart failure.
- *Functional capacity*: Observational clues such as shortness of breath while speaking or walking into the clinic.
- *Other systems*: Neurologic baseline, signs of malnutrition or frailty, and peripheral vascular disease.

7.3 Functional Capacity and METs

Functional capacity reflects the ability of the cardiovascular and pulmonary systems to meet metabolic demands during stress and exertion. Surgical procedures impose a physiologic burden similar to moderate to high-intensity exercise. Patients with poor exercise tolerance are less able to compensate, predisposing them to cardiac ischemia, hypoxemia, and hemodynamic instability.

7.3.1 Physiology of Functional Capacity

- *Oxygen delivery (DO_2)* depends on cardiac output, hemoglobin concentration, and oxygen saturation.
- *Oxygen consumption (VO_2)* rises with activity; maximal VO_2 is a predictor of survival across cardiovascular diseases.
- *METs* translate activity-related oxygen consumption into a standardized unit: 1 MET = 3.5 mL O_2/kg/min (resting metabolic rate of a 40-year-old, 70-kg man).

7.4 METs and Daily Activities

Functional capacity is estimated by correlating self-reported ability to perform activities with known MET values. Examples of MET values are presented in Table 7.1.

Table 7.1 Examples of activities by MET level

METs	Example activities
1–2	Eating, dressing, walking indoors
3–4	Walking up a hill, climbing one flight of stairs, heavy housework
5–6	Dancing, gardening, brisk walking at 4 mph
≥7	Jogging, swimming laps, playing singles tennis

7.5 Risk Stratification Using METs

- *≥4 METs*: Generally adequate reserve; low risk for most non-cardiac surgeries.
- *<4 METs*: Increased perioperative risk, especially for major vascular or thoracic surgery.
- In patients with poor functional capacity and multiple risk factors, further testing should be considered (e.g., stress imaging and cardiopulmonary exercise testing).

7.6 ASA Physical Status Classification

- The American Society of Anesthesiologists (ASA) Physical Status (PS) Classification System provides a standardized framework to communicate baseline health and surgical risk:
  - *ASA I*: Healthy patient, no systemic disease (e.g., young, non-smoking, healthy adult).
  - *ASA II*: Mild systemic disease without functional limitation (e.g., well-controlled hypertension, diabetes without end-organ damage, and mild asthma).
  - *ASA III*: Severe systemic disease with substantive functional limitation (e.g., poorly controlled diabetes or hypertension, stable angina, and chronic obstructive pulmonary disease (COPD) with daily symptoms).
  - *ASA IV*: Severe systemic disease that is a constant threat to life (e.g., recent myocardial infarction, decompensated heart failure, and severe valve disease)
  - *ASA V*: Moribund patient not expected to survive without surgery (e.g., ruptured abdominal aortic aneurysm with shock).
  - *ASA VI*: Brain-dead patient undergoing organ procurement.
  - An "E" suffix (e.g., *ASA II-E*) is added for emergency surgery.
- Although ASA Physical Status Classification is subjective, it correlates with perioperative morbidity and mortality. It remains one of the simplest and most widely used tools for risk stratification, easily understood across surgical and medical teams. Surgery-related risk of major complications is presented in Table 7.2.
- Table 7.2. Surgical Risk Stratification by Estimated 30-Day Major Adverse Cardiac Event (MACE) Risk.

Table 7.2 Surgical risk stratification by estimated 30-day MACE risk

Risk category	Estimated 30-day cardiac risk	Examples of surgical procedures
High-risk surgery (>5% risk of MACE)	>5%	Major vascular surgery (open aortic or peripheral vascular surgery) Thoracic surgery (esophagectomy, pneumonectomy) Liver transplant or major hepatic resection Major pancreatic surgery Emergency major abdominal surgery (perforated viscus, bowel ischemia)
Intermediate-risk surgery (1–5% risk of MACE)	1–5%	Carotid endarterectomy Head and neck surgery Intraperitoneal or intrathoracic procedures (non-major) Orthopedic surgery (hip/knee replacement, spine surgery) Prostate surgery
Low-risk surgery (<1% risk of MACE)	<1%	Cataract surgery Superficial dermatologic surgery Breast surgery Endoscopic procedures (colonoscopy, bronchoscopy) Ambulatory dental procedures

7.7 Risk Stratification

The 2024 AHA/ACC perioperative guidelines outline a stepwise algorithm:

1. *Determine urgency of surgery*: Emergent surgery (e.g., trauma, ruptured aneurysm, type A aortic dissection, etc.) may preclude formal optimization.
2. *Identify active cardiac conditions*: Unstable angina, decompensated heart failure, severe arrhythmias, or severe valvular disease warrant postponement until stabilization.
3. *Estimate surgical risk*: High-risk procedures (e.g., major vascular, intrathoracic, or intra-abdominal surgery) carry greater physiological stress (see Table 7.1).
4. *Assess functional capacity*: >4 METs of activity indicates lower risk; poor or unknown functional status may warrant additional evaluation.
5. *Use validated risk calculators*: Such as the Revised Cardiac Risk Index (RCRI), the National Surgical Quality Improvement Program (NSQIP) Surgical Risk Calculator (https://riskcalculator.facs.org/RiskCalculator/PatientInfo.jsp), or disease-specific indices. RCRI (https://www.mdcalc.com/calc/1739/revised-cardiac-risk-index-pre-operative-risk) is presented in Table 7.3.

Table 7.3 Revised Cardiac Risk Index

Risk factor	Points	Total RCRI score	Estimated risk of MACE
High-risk surgery (intraperitoneal, intrathoracic, or suprainguinal vascular)	1	0	~0.4%
History of ischemic heart disease	1	1	~0.9%
History of congestive heart failure	1	2	~6.6%
History of cerebrovascular disease (stroke or TIA)	1	≥3	>11%
Insulin-treated diabetes mellitus	1	–	–
Preoperative serum creatinine >2.0 mg/dL (177 μmol/L)	1	–	–

Reported cardiac complications include: cardiac death, myocardial infarction, complete heart block, pulmonary edema or cardiac arrest

6. *Consider biomarker testing*: The 2024 guideline expands the role of natriuretic peptides (brain natriuretic peptide (BNP)/N-terminal pro brain natriuretic peptide (NT-proBNP)) and troponins for patients at elevated risk undergoing major surgery.
7. *Pursue further testing only if results would change management*: Stress testing or echocardiography is not recommended routinely, but may be reasonable if functional capacity is poor and surgical risk is high.

This stepwise approach discourages indiscriminate testing, emphasizing individualized, evidence-based evaluation.

7.8 Special Considerations

7.8.1 Valvular Heart Disease

- Severe symptomatic aortic stenosis remains a high-risk lesion. Elective noncardiac surgery should generally be deferred until valve intervention.
- Severe mitral stenosis or regurgitation also confers elevated risk, particularly in the setting of atrial fibrillation or pulmonary hypertension.

7.8.2 Heart Failure

Decompensated heart failure carries a very high perioperative risk. Patients should be optimized medically, and elective procedures deferred until euvolemia and stability are achieved.

7.8.3 Coronary Artery Disease (CAD)

- Patients with recent acute coronary syndrome or percutaneous coronary intervention (PCI) require individualized planning.
- Timing of noncardiac surgery after PCI remains critical:
  - Bare-metal stent: ≥30 days.
  - Drug-eluting stent: ideally ≥6 months, minimum 3 months if urgent surgery is required.
- Dual antiplatelet therapy interruption should be avoided when possible. Consultation with the cardiology service is often needed.

7.8.4 Arrhythmias and Devices

Preoperative interrogation of pacemakers and implantable cardioverter-defibrillators (ICDs) is essential. Perioperative management may require temporary reprogramming or magnet application to prevent inappropriate ICD therapies or pacemaker malfunction during electrocautery use. Because magnet response is device-specific and can be unpredictable if not previously confirmed, reliance on magnets is less desirable. Ideally, devices should be formally reprogrammed before surgery and restored to baseline settings postoperatively.

7.8.5 Pulmonary Disease

COPD, asthma, and obstructive sleep apnea increase the risk of postoperative pulmonary complications. Optimization includes bronchodilator therapy, smoking cessation, and continuous positive airway pressure (CPAP) adherence.

Respiratory complications such as pneumonia, atelectasis, and respiratory failure are among the most common causes of perioperative morbidity. Risk is increased in patients with COPD, OSA, obesity, and poor functional status. Several validated tools aid in risk prediction, including the ARISCAT score (https://www.mdcalc.com/calc/10022/ariscat-score-postoperative-pulmonary-complications) and the Gupta Postoperative Respiratory Failure Risk Calculator (https://www.mdcalc.com/calc/10193/gupta-postoperative-respiratory-failure-risk), which combine clinical and procedural variables to guide perioperative planning.

7.8.6 Renal and Hepatic Disease

Chronic kidney disease increases the risk of fluid overload, electrolyte disturbances, and impaired drug clearance. Advanced liver disease carries risks of bleeding, encephalopathy, and hemodynamic instability, warranting multidisciplinary planning.

7.8.7 Pulmonary Arterial Hypertension (PAH)

Patients with PAH face markedly elevated perioperative risk, with mortality rates reported as high as 7–10% in noncardiac surgery. The major concerns are right ventricular failure, arrhythmias, hypoxemia, and hemodynamic collapse in response to anesthesia, mechanical ventilation, or surgical stress. General anesthesia, positive pressure ventilation, hypoxia, hypercarbia, and acidosis can all increase pulmonary vascular resistance, precipitating decompensation. Perioperative planning includes:

- Preoperative optimization with PAH-specific therapies (endothelin receptor antagonists, PDE-5 inhibitors, prostacyclin analogues). Preprocedural consultation with the physician managing PAH is essential.
- Careful intraoperative monitoring, often with invasive hemodynamics.
- Maintenance of sinus rhythm, normoxia, and normocapnia.
- Avoidance of systemic hypotension, as the RV depends on adequate coronary perfusion pressure.
- Elective surgery in severe PAH should be approached cautiously, ideally in tertiary centers with anesthesia, cardiology, and critical care expertise.

7.9 Nothing by Mouth (NPO) (Fasting) Guidelines and Aspiration Risk (Adults)

- Adherence to fasting guidelines reduces aspiration risk. Elective procedures are typically canceled if NPO instructions are not followed (see Table 7.4 for more information). For urgent/emergent surgery, anesthesiologists will typically proceed with rapid sequence induction (RSI) to secure the airway promptly (RSI is often not ideal in this context because of its association with hemodynamic instability, risk of hypoxemia, and intraoperative awareness due to potential underdosing of sedative agents, among other concerns). Certain populations are considered "full stomach" regardless of reported fasting times—notably trauma, pregnancy, small bowel obstruction, and critically ill patients.

Table 7.4 Recommended adult NPO times

Ingested material	Minimum fasting period	Examples
Clear liquids	2 hours	Water, apple juice, black coffee/tea (no milk)
Breast milk	4 hours	–
Infant formula/nonhuman milk	6 hours	Standard formula, cow's milk
Light meal	6 hours	Toast, fruit, non-fatty foods
Fatty/fried meal or meat	≥8 hours	Burgers, steak, fried/greasy meals

7.10 Perioperative Medication Management

Medication reconciliation is central to preoperative evaluation. While a comprehensive discussion is beyond the scope of this chapter, several key drug classes warrant emphasis:

- *Antiplatelet agents and anticoagulants*:
  - Aspirin is often continued in patients with coronary stents or high cardiovascular risk.
  - P2Y12 inhibitors (clopidogrel, ticagrelor, and prasugrel) are usually continued for recent stents; otherwise, interruption requires balancing bleeding versus thrombotic risk.
  - Perioperative bridging decisions require individualized planning. The active use of antithrombotic agents, except for aspirin, generally precludes patients from receiving neuraxial anesthesia and certain regional anesthesia techniques.
  - Certain procedures carry a particularly high risk of catastrophic bleeding in closed, confined spaces, where even a small hemorrhage can cause major morbidity. For these surgeries, continuation of anticoagulants or antiplatelets is usually avoided unless the thrombotic risk is extreme:
  - *Neurosurgery (intracranial or spinal)*: Even minor bleeding can lead to devastating complications such as hematoma, spinal cord compression, or intracranial hemorrhage.
  - *Ophthalmic surgery (intraocular, especially posterior chamber)*: Intraocular bleeding may cause irreversible vision loss.
  - *Inner ear surgery*: Hemorrhage in the labyrinthine structures can impair hearing and balance permanently.
  - In these cases, the balance of risk generally favors temporary interruption of anticoagulation/antiplatelet therapy, with individualized planning and coordination among surgeons, anesthesiologists, and internists/cardiologists. Bridging strategies may be considered if thrombotic risk is high.
- *Beta-blockers*:
  - Should be continued perioperatively if the patient is already taking them.
  - Initiation shortly before surgery is not recommended due to the risk of bradycardia and hypotension.
- *Angiotensin converting enzyme (ACE) inhibitors/Angiotensin receptor blocker (ARBs)*:
  - Continuation is debated. Some guidelines suggest holding the morning of surgery to avoid difficult-to-treat hypotension, particularly in the setting of general anesthesia.
  - Continuation may be reasonable in patients with heart failure and reduced ejection fraction or difficult-to-treat hypertension.

7.10.1 Glucocorticoids (Steroids)

Patients receiving chronic glucocorticoid therapy or who are otherwise at risk of hypothalamic–pituitary–adrenal axis suppression require special consideration in the perioperative period. The primary concern is adrenal insufficiency and hemodynamic collapse when patients are unable to mount an adequate cortisol response to surgical stress.

- *Who is at risk*:
  - Patients taking the equivalent of prednisone ≥5 mg daily for ≥3 weeks.
  - Patients with clinical features of Cushing's syndrome.
  - Recent high-dose glucocorticoid exposure within the past year.
- *Stress-dose steroid indications*:
  - Required for moderate to major surgical stress in patients at risk of adrenal suppression.
  - Minor procedures under local/regional anesthesia typically do not require supplementation.
- *Typical regimens*:
  - *Minor surgery (e.g., inguinal hernia repair)*: Continue baseline dose; often no supplementation needed.
  - *Moderate surgery (e.g., joint replacement, abdominal hysterectomy)*: Hydrocortisone 50 mg IV at induction, then 25 mg IV every 8 hours for 24 hours; resume baseline dose thereafter.
  - *Major surgery (e.g., cardiac, thoracic, major vascular, and abdominal surgery)*: Hydrocortisone 100 mg IV at induction and then 50 mg IV every 8 hours for 24–48 hours; taper rapidly to baseline as patient stabilizes.
- *Tapering*:
  - After the stress period, reduce steroids back to the patient's baseline regimen as soon as clinically feasible.
  - Prolonged high-dose "stress coverage" is unnecessary and increases risks of infection, hyperglycemia, and impaired wound healing.

7.11 Laboratory and Diagnostic Testing

Routine testing without indication is discouraged. Targeted evaluation should be based on clinical context:

- *ECG*: Reasonable for patients with known CAD, arrhythmias, or significant structural heart disease undergoing moderate/high-risk surgery.
- *Echocardiography*: In patients with known cardiac or valvular disease, repeat transthoracic echocardiography is generally reasonable when prior imaging is outdated or no longer reflective of the current clinical state. For known moderate to severe valvular heart disease, repeat echocardiography is appropriate if no study has been performed within the preceding 12 months, or sooner if there has

been any change in symptoms, functional capacity, or physical examination findings. For mild valvular disease or stable cardiomyopathy, repeat imaging is typically reasonable if the last study is older than 2–3 years, particularly in patients undergoing intermediate- or high-risk surgery. In all cases, earlier reassessment is warranted with new or worsening dyspnea, signs of heart failure, arrhythmia, or changes in murmur intensity, as these findings may indicate disease progression with important perioperative implications.
- *BNP or troponin*: It is reasonable to obtain these biomarkers in patients at elevated cardiovascular risk who are undergoing high-risk surgery, particularly if the results are expected to influence perioperative management or the anesthetic plan.
- *Chest radiography*: Not recommended routinely; indicated for unexplained cardiopulmonary symptoms.

7.12 Shared Decision-Making and Patient Engagement

Modern preoperative evaluation emphasizes not only risk stratification but also communication. Shared decision-making involves:

- Informing patients of perioperative risks in understandable terms
- Discussing how comorbidities influence outcomes
- Aligning perioperative strategies with patient preferences, especially in frail or elderly patients, where surgical benefit may be marginal

Internists, who often have longstanding relationships with patients, are uniquely positioned to facilitate these conversations and integrate patient values into perioperative planning.

7.13 Conclusion

Preoperative assessment and optimization are critical to safe surgical care. Contemporary approaches—guided by the 2024 AHA/ACC/ACS/SCA framework—emphasize individualized evaluation, selective testing, coordinated medication management, adherence to NPO fasting protocols, and thoughtful planning for high-risk populations. Internists and anesthesiologists share responsibility for risk stratification, comorbidity optimization, and patient counseling. Collaborative, evidence-based preoperative evaluation improves safety, outcomes, and the patient experience.

Key Takeaways

1. Preoperative assessment aims to identify risk, optimize comorbidities, and support shared decision-making.
2. Functional capacity (>4 METs) strongly predicts surgical tolerance; poor capacity warrants targeted testing (e.g., cardiopulmonary exercise testing and stress imaging).
3. ASA-PS, RCRI, and NSQIP remain core frameworks for standardized risk stratification.
4. High-risk populations (valvular disease, heart failure, PAH, and major end-organ dysfunction) require individualized, multidisciplinary plans.
5. Modern practice emphasizes selective testing, coordinated medication management, and strict NPO adherence; elective cases are canceled if noncompliant, and urgent cases proceed with RSI, with certain groups treated as full stomach regardless of fasting times.

Suggested Reading

1. Thompson A, Fleischmann KE, Smilowitz NR, et al. 2024 AHA/ACC/ACS/ASNC/HRS/SCA/SCCT/SCMR/SVM guideline for perioperative cardiovascular management for noncardiac surgery: a report of the American College of Cardiology/American Heart Association Joint Committee on Clinical Practice Guidelines. Circulation. 2024;150(19):e351–442.
2. https://www.asahq.org/standards-and-practice-parameters/statement-on-asa-physical-status-classification-system.
3. Lee TH, Marcantonio ER, Mangione CM, et al. Derivation and prospective validation of a simple index for prediction of cardiac risk of major noncardiac surgery. Circulation. 1999;100(10):1043–9.
4. Gupta PK, Gupta H, Sundaram A, et al. Development and validation of a risk calculator for prediction of cardiac risk after surgery. Circulation. 2011;124(4):381–7.
5. Wright DE, Knuesel SJ, Nagarur A, et al. Examining risk: a systematic review of perioperative cardiac risk prediction indices. Mayo Clin Proc. 2019;94(11):2277–90.
6. Myers J, Prakash M, Froelicher V, et al. Exercise capacity and mortality among men referred for exercise testing. N Engl J Med. 2002;346(11):793–801.
7. Wijeysundera DN, Pearse RM, Shulman MA, et al. Assessment of functional capacity before major non-cardiac surgery: an international, prospective cohort study. Lancet. 2018;391(10140):2631–40.
8. Devereaux PJ, Sessler DI. Cardiac complications in patients undergoing major noncardiac surgery. N Engl J Med. 2015;373(23):2258–69.
9. Rajagopal S, Ruetzler K, Ghadimi K, et al. Evaluation and management of pulmonary hypertension in noncardiac surgery: a scientific statement from the American Heart Association. Circulation. 2023;147(17):1317–43.
10. Sameed M, Choi H, Auron M, et al. Preoperative pulmonary risk assessment. Respir Care. 2021;66(7):1150–66.
11. Practice guidelines for preoperative fasting and the use of pharmacologic agents to reduce the risk of pulmonary aspiration: application to healthy patients undergoing elective procedures: an updated report by the American Society of Anesthesiologists Task Force on preoperative fasting and the use of pharmacologic agents to reduce the risk of pulmonary aspiration. Anesthesiology. 2017;126(3):376–93.
12. Robinson M, Davidson A. Aspiration under anaesthesia: risk assessment and decision-making. Contin Educ Anaesth Crit Care Pain. 2014;14(4):171–5.

8 The Role of the Internist in Perioperative Medicine

8.1 Introduction

Perioperative medicine lies at the intersection of surgery, anesthesiology, and internal medicine. The internist's role is pivotal in ensuring that patients undergoing surgery are properly evaluated, optimized, and supported across the perioperative continuum, whereas anesthesiologists focus on intraoperative management and surgical teams on procedural success, internists bring longitudinal knowledge of the patient's medical history, comorbidities, and functional status.

The American Heart Association (AHA) and American College of Cardiology (ACC) guidelines on perioperative evaluation emphasize a collaborative, stepwise approach. Within this framework, internists are uniquely positioned to identify and manage medical risks, to advise on the timing and appropriateness of surgery, and to align perioperative care with the patient's overall health trajectory.

It is important, however, to clarify the scope of the internist's contribution. Recommendations should focus on whether the patient is medically optimized, what steps can further aid in optimization, and what general risks remain if surgery proceeds. While internists occasionally attempt to advise on anesthetic technique (e.g., recommending regional anesthesia, advising against hypotension, or suggesting that a cardiac anesthesiologist is "required"), such comments fall outside the internist's domain. These statements, while well-intentioned, are often unhelpful because they do not reflect the nuanced physiological trade-offs, surgical considerations, or anesthetic expertise required for intraoperative decision-making. Instead, anesthesiologists prefer concise, actionable input about medical optimization and residual risk.

This chapter explores the appropriate role of the internist in perioperative medicine, highlighting three domains: risk stratification, medical optimization, and effective communication with anesthesia colleagues.

A. Mirrakhimov, *Anesthesiology Demystified for the Internist*,
https://doi.org/10.1007/978-3-032-16811-5_8

8.2 Preoperative Risk Stratification

8.2.1 Purpose of Risk Stratification

Risk stratification is not about eliminating all risk, which is often an impossible task, but rather about quantifying risk, identifying opportunities for optimization, and supporting informed decision-making by the patient, surgeon, and anesthesiologist. Internists contribute by bringing deep familiarity with comorbid conditions and the patient's functional baseline.

8.2.2 Frameworks for Cardiac Risk

The 2024 AHA/ACC perioperative guidelines recommend a stepwise approach (see Chap. 7 for more information):

1. *Surgical urgency*: Emergent cases often proceed with minimal evaluation, while elective procedures allow time for optimization.
2. *Active cardiac conditions*: Unstable angina, decompensated heart failure, severe valvular disease, or significant arrhythmias warrant stabilization before surgery.
3. *Surgical risk*: Procedures are classified as high, intermediate, or low risk for major adverse cardiac events (MACEs).
4. *Functional capacity*: Typically assessed by metabolic equivalent (METs) or duke activity status index (DASI) questionnaire; <4 METs indicates increased risk.
5. *Risk calculators*: Tools such as the Revised Cardiac Risk Index (RCRI) or National Surgical Quality Improvement Program (NSQIP) calculators provide structured estimates.
6. *Biomarkers*: Natriuretic peptides and troponins may further refine risk in some complex cases.

Internists should be familiar with these frameworks and apply them judiciously, always asking: Will additional testing change management or surgical decision-making?

8.2.3 Pulmonary and Other Risks

Beyond cardiac evaluation, internists help anticipate pulmonary complications (e.g., pneumonia and respiratory failure), which are among the most common perioperative morbidities. Tools such as ARISCAT or NSQIP respiratory risk calculators can assist. Internists also stratify risks associated with renal disease, hepatic dysfunction, frailty, and hematologic conditions.

8.2.4 The Internist's Deliverable

The internist's task is not to declare whether surgery should or should not occur, but rather to provide:

- An estimate of risk (low, intermediate, or high, ideally quantified)
- A description of modifiable versus non-modifiable risk factors
- Clear documentation of any conditions that require optimization prior to proceeding

This information empowers the surgeon and anesthesiologist to make appropriate intraoperative and perioperative decisions.

8.3 Medical Optimization

8.3.1 Cardiovascular Optimization

- *Heart failure*: Ensure euvolemia, optimize guideline-directed therapy, and delay elective procedures in decompensated cases.
- *Ischemic heart disease*: Manage angina, assess stent history, and ensure appropriate antiplatelet therapy.
- *Arrhythmias*: Rate or rhythm control, anticoagulation management, and device interrogation when indicated.

8.3.2 Pulmonary Optimization

- *COPD and asthma*: Reinforce inhaler adherence, consider preoperative steroids if unstable, and encourage smoking cessation.
- *OSA*: Reinforce CPAP use and notify perioperative team.

8.3.3 Renal Optimization

- Adjust medication dosing for estimated glomerular filtration rate (eGFR), ensure euvolemia, and plan dialysis around surgical timing if applicable.

8.3.4 Endocrine and Metabolic Optimization

- *Diabetes*: Aim for reasonable glycemic control, often targeting HbA1c <8%. Manage perioperative insulin regimens.
- *Thyroid disease*: Avoid elective surgery in patients with untreated severe hyperthyroidism or myxedema coma.

- *Adrenal suppression*: Identify patients at risk and plan for perioperative stress-dose steroids.

8.3.5 Hematologic and Antithrombotic Considerations

Internists play a critical role in managing anticoagulation and antiplatelet therapy, balancing thrombotic and bleeding risks. Certain surgeries (e.g., neurosurgery, ophthalmic, and inner ear) usually mandate interruption due to catastrophic bleeding risk in closed spaces, whereas others may safely proceed with continuation. Coordination with surgeons, anesthesiologists, and cardiologists is essential.

8.3.6 Infectious Disease and Nutrition

Active infection should be treated before elective surgery. Malnutrition and frailty predict poor outcomes; nutritional supplementation and physical prehabilitation may reduce complications.

8.4 Communication and Handoffs with Anesthesia

8.4.1 Principles of Effective Communication

Consultation notes should be concise, structured, and actionable. The anesthesiology team wants to know:

1. Is the patient medically optimized?
2. What steps remain for optimization, if any?
3. What general risks remain if surgery proceeds?

This information helps anesthesiologists plan intraoperative care and informs discussions with the surgical team and patient.

8.4.2 What Anesthesiologists Do Not Find Helpful

Out of respect for professional boundaries, internists should avoid recommendations outside their scope. For example:

- Advising on the mode of anesthesia (e.g., "regional preferred"): The choice of general versus regional anesthesia depends on surgical, technical, and patient-specific factors best judged by anesthesiologists.

- Recommending hemodynamic targets (e.g., "avoid hypotension"): Anesthesiologists continuously balance blood pressure, perfusion, and surgical requirements. Stating the obvious is not actionable.
- Suggesting which anesthesiologist (e.g., cardiac trained) should provide care: Staffing decisions reflect institutional structures and should not be dictated by consultants.

Such statements, though well-meaning, are often perceived as intrusive. Far more valuable is clear documentation that the patient is optimized from a medical perspective, with delineation of residual risks.

8.4.3 What Is Helpful

Instead, internists should:

- Document comorbidity status (e.g., "congestive heart failure (CHF) compensated, last BNP 120, no edema").
- Highlight unresolved issues (e.g., "Recent angina, cardiology evaluation pending").
- Clarify medication management (e.g., "Continue beta-blocker, hold ACE-I morning of surgery").
- Provide risk stratification using validated frameworks (e.g., "RCRI = 2, ~6.6% risk of MACE").
- State overall impression (e.g., "Medically optimized, elevated cardiac risk, but no active contraindication to proceeding").

This style of communication supports anesthesiologists in making technical and intraoperative decisions while preserving the internist's essential role as a perioperative consultant.

8.5 Conclusion

The role of the internist in perioperative medicine is indispensable. By focusing on risk stratification, medical optimization, and clear communication, internists enhance patient safety, support anesthesiologists and surgeons, and facilitate informed patient decisions.

Importantly, recommendations should remain within the internist's expertise: describing comorbidities, optimization strategies, and residual risks. Advising on anesthetic technique, intraoperative hemodynamic targets, or personnel assignments is unnecessary and often counterproductive. A respectful, collaborative approach ensures that each specialty contributes its unique expertise, reinforcing the shared mission of safe, patient-centered care.

Key Takeaways

1. Scope-appropriate deliverable: Quantify risk, list modifiable versus non-modifiable factors, outline optimization steps, and provide medication plans—avoid dictating anesthetic technique or intraoperative targets.
2. Structured risk assessment: Apply stepwise frameworks (urgency → active conditions → surgical risk → functional capacity → calculators/biomarkers) and test only when results change management.
3. Targeted optimization: Stabilize heart failure (HF)/coronary artery disease (CAD)/arrhythmias, treat pulmonary disease and OSA, adjust for chronic kidney disease/cirrhosis, address diabetes/thyroid/adrenal issues, and plan perioperative anticoagulation/antiplatelets.
4. Anticipate noncardiac complications: Use tools for pulmonary risk, promote prehabilitation and infection control, and manage nutrition/frailty to reduce morbidity.
5. Communicate effectively: Provide concise, actionable notes and collaborate with anesthesia and surgery to align plans with patient goals via shared decision-making.

Suggested Reading

1. Thompson A, Fleischmann KE, Smilowitz NR, et al. 2024 AHA/ACC/ACS/ASNC/HRS/SCA/SCCT/SCMR/SVM guideline for perioperative cardiovascular management for noncardiac surgery: a report of the American College of Cardiology/American Heart Association Joint Committee on clinical practice guidelines. Circulation. 2024;150(19):e351–442.
2. Pausjenssen L, Ward HA, Card SE. An internist's role in perioperative medicine: a survey of surgeons' opinions. BMC Fam Pract. 2008;9:4.
3. Shaw M, Pelecanos AM, Mudge AM. Evaluation of internal medicine physician or multidisciplinary team comanagement of surgical patients and clinical outcomes: a systematic review and meta-analysis. JAMA Netw Open. 2020;3(5):e204088.
4. Osborne AF, Aung AK, Johnson D, et al. General physicians and perioperative medicine. What is on the horizon? Intern Med J. 2024;54(1):12–5.
5. Adesanya AO, Joshi GP. Hospitalists and anesthesiologists as perioperative physicians: are their roles complementary? Proc (Bayl Univ Med Cent). 2007;20(2):140–2.
6. Lubarsky D, Candiotti K. Giving anesthesiologists what they want: how to write a useful preoperative consult. Cleve Clin J Med. 2009;76(Suppl 4):S32–6.
7. Wijeysundera DN. Preoperative consultations by anesthesiologists. Curr Opin Anaesthesiol. 2011;24(3):326–30.

Perioperative Testing from the Lens of Anesthesiologists

9

9.1 Introduction

Preoperative evaluation is a cornerstone of perioperative medicine. While internists often focus on long-term management of chronic disease, anesthesiologists view preoperative testing through a distinct lens—one that emphasizes immediate perioperative risk, induction strategy, intraoperative monitoring, and safe recovery. Surgery and anesthesia impose substantial physiological stress on the patient. Patients may experience hypovolemia, acute blood loss, cardiac arrhythmia, ischemia, and shifts in acid–base or electrolyte status.

Consequently, anesthesiologists interpret common laboratory and imaging studies not simply as background data, but as tools to anticipate intraoperative events, choose anesthetic techniques, and define monitoring and resuscitation goals. This chapter reviews key perioperative tests, including complete blood count (CBC), comprehensive metabolic panel (CMP), type and screen (T&S), coagulation studies, electrocardiogram (ECG), and echocardiography, from the anesthesiologist's perspective.

9.2 General Principles of Perioperative Testing

Professional societies emphasize that perioperative testing should be selective and clinically guided, not routine. The American Society of Anesthesiologists and American College of Cardiology/American Heart Association recommend testing when it is expected to influence management. Nevertheless, anesthesiologists often find value in tests that may not alter long-term internist decision-making but carry implications for anesthetic induction, airway planning, intraoperative monitoring, and transfusion readiness.

A. Mirrakhimov, *Anesthesiology Demystified for the Internist*,
https://doi.org/10.1007/978-3-032-16811-5_9

9.3 Complete Blood Count

9.3.1 Hemoglobin and Hematocrit

From the anesthesiologist's perspective, hemoglobin (Hb) and hematocrit (Hct) levels inform oxygen-carrying capacity, transfusion thresholds, and risk tolerance for blood loss.

- A patient with a baseline hemoglobin of 9 g/dL who is scheduled for a Whipple procedure—a major operation performed for resectable pancreatic, duodenal, or biliary malignancies—requires a different transfusion strategy than a patient with a baseline hemoglobin of 14 g/dL.
- Even if internists deem moderate anemia acceptable for outpatient management, anesthesiologists may alter induction drugs, prepare blood products, or request invasive monitoring when anticipating large blood loss.

9.3.2 White Blood Cell Count

An elevated white blood cell count may indicate an underlying infection, increasing the risk of sepsis and hemodynamic instability during induction or intraoperative management. This is particularly relevant in patients undergoing procedures such as endoscopic retrograde cholangiopancreatography for cholangitis or urgent ureteral stent placement, where instrumentation can precipitate a transient worsening of the hemodynamic profile or even profound cardiovascular instability. Severe neutropenia may necessitate protective isolation, increase the risk of surgical site infection, and require the use of stricter aseptic techniques. It also warrants avoiding certain monitoring devices (e.g., rectal temperature probes) and raises concerns regarding impaired wound healing.

9.3.3 Platelet Count

Platelets are critical for hemostasis.

- Counts below 100,000/μL prompt anesthesiologists to consider neuraxial anesthesia risks.
- Counts <50,000/μL often preclude neuraxial and certain regional anesthesia techniques (e.g. paravertebral nerve block) techniques and may increase bleeding risk during airway manipulation or invasive line placement.

9.4 Comprehensive Metabolic Panel

9.4.1 Electrolytes

- *Potassium*: Dyskalemia increases the risk of perioperative arrhythmias. For example, the neuromuscular blocker succinylcholine should be used with extreme caution—if at all—in patients with baseline hyperkalemia, as it can cause a transient rise in serum potassium, further exacerbating the condition and predisposing to life-threatening arrhythmias.
- *Sodium*: Severe hyponatremia can precipitate seizures under surgical stress (which can be masked under general anesthesia).
- *Calcium and Magnesium*: Perturbations affect neuromuscular blocker responses and arrhythmia risk.

9.4.2 Renal Function

Blood urea nitrogen (BUN) and creatinine levels help anesthesiologists:

- Adjust dosing of renally cleared drugs (e.g., neuromuscular blockers and some opioids).
- Prepare for perioperative dialysis coordination in end stage renal disease (ESRD) patients.

9.4.3 Hepatic Function

Liver enzymes and bilirubin are interpreted for:

- Coagulation risk (via synthetic dysfunction)
- Drug metabolism (reduced clearance of opioids, benzodiazepines, dexmedetomidine, or muscle relaxants)
- Risk of encephalopathy postoperatively

9.5 Type and Screen

9.5.1 Importance for Anesthesiologists

Anesthesiologists rely heavily on T&S for anticipating and managing blood loss.

- Even procedures expected to have "minimal" bleeding may be catastrophic if an uncontrolled hemorrhage occurs.
- Crossmatched blood may be prepared for high-risk surgeries (e.g., cardiac, liver resection, and trauma), while a simple T&S may suffice for lower-risk procedures.

9.5.2 Key Considerations

- Patients with multiple transfusions or alloimmunization may require special matching, necessitating early coordination with the blood bank.
- Anesthesiologists also integrate T&S into massive transfusion protocols, ensuring rapid product availability in emergencies.

9.6 Coagulation Studies (Prothrombin Time (PT)/International Normalized Ratio (INR), Activated Partial Thromboplastin Time (aPTT), Fibrinogen)

9.6.1 Why They Matter for Anesthesiologists

Abnormal coagulation results guide anesthetic planning:

- *Neuraxial anesthesia*: Contraindicated in the presence of coagulopathy.
- *Intraoperative bleeding risk*: Impacts transfusion strategies and the need for antifibrinolytic agents (e.g., tranexamic acid).
- *Induction planning*: Patients with coagulopathy may have tenuous hemodynamics requiring gentle induction to avoid catastrophic bleeding or hemodynamic collapse.

9.6.2 Special Considerations

- *Direct oral anticoagulant (DOACs) and antiplatelet agents*: Routine laboratory studies may not fully capture the complexities of coagulation abnormalities. As a result, anesthesiologists often obtain additional tests, such as viscoelastic assays [e.g., thromboelastography (TEG) or rotational thromboelastometry (ROTEM)], to gain a more nuanced and dynamic assessment of a patient's coagulation profile.
- *Liver disease patients*: May show abnormal PT/INR, but anesthesiologists interpret results in the context of overall hemostatic balance, not simply numbers.

9.7 Additional Laboratory Tests

1. *Arterial blood gas with lactate*
   - *Why useful for anesthesiologists*:
     - Provides baseline oxygenation, ventilation, and acid–base status.
     - Guides induction strategy in patients with hypoxemia, hypercapnia, or metabolic acidosis.
     - Elevated lactate may suggest poor perfusion or occult sepsis—critical for intraoperative vigilance.
   - *Typical context*: Severe chronic obstructive pulmonary disease (COPD), interstitial lung disease, sepsis, trauma, or liver failure.

2. *Venous blood gas with co-oximetry*
    - Allows screening of pH, CO_2, and lactate when arterial sampling is not yet obtained or available.
    - Co-oximetry can identify carbon monoxide or methemoglobinemia exposures—important in smoke inhalation or toxicology cases.
3. *Blood glucose and HbA1c*
    - Internists use HbA1c for chronic glycemic control; anesthesiologists focus more on perioperative glucose since both hypo- and hyperglycemia affect neurologic recovery, wound healing, and infection risk.
4. *Pregnancy testing (β-hCG)*
    - Required for women of childbearing age for medicolegal and safety reasons.
    - Informs anesthetic drug selection (teratogenic risk), airway considerations, and monitoring for aspiration risk.
5. *Thyroid function tests*
    - Rarely obtained preoperatively unless clinical suspicion exists.
    - *Why relevant for anesthesiologists*: Severe untreated hyperthyroidism increases risk of thyroid storm; hypothyroidism may alter drug metabolism and hemodynamic stability.
6. *Brain natriuretic peptide (BNP)/NT-pro-BNP*
    - Used increasingly in perioperative risk stratification (especially noncardiac surgery in patients with suspected heart failure).
    - For anesthesiologists, elevated BNP suggests vulnerability to fluid shifts and perioperative cardiac events, guiding monitoring intensity.
7. *Viscoelastic Testing (TEG/ROTEM)*
    - Provides dynamic clot formation profiles.
    - Valuable in liver transplantation, cardiac surgery, trauma, and obstetric hemorrhage, where standard INR/PTT may not predict bleeding risk accurately.

9.8 Electrocardiogram

9.8.1 Baseline Reference

Internists may view ECGs primarily as diagnostic for ischemia or arrhythmias. Anesthesiologists, however, also value them as baseline comparators for intraoperative monitoring and postoperative care.

- A known left bundle branch block prevents misinterpretation of intraoperative ST-segment changes.
- Pre-existing atrial fibrillation informs perioperative rate control strategies and monitoring for embolic complications.

9.8.2 Risk Stratification

Anesthesiologists use ECGs to:

- Anticipate intraoperative arrhythmias under volatile agents or during electrolyte shifts.
- Plan for pacing capability in patients with conduction disease.
- Consider pre-induction anti-arrhythmic strategies in high-risk cases.

9.9 Echocardiography

9.9.1 Role in Perioperative Planning

Echocardiography is invaluable for anesthesiologists, even when it may not alter internist management. Surgery and anesthesia are major physiologic stressors, and echocardiographic findings guide induction goals, hemodynamic targets, and intraoperative monitoring.

Some Examples:

- *Severe aortic stenosis*: Anesthetic induction and intraoperative management should be guided by the principles of maintaining hemodynamic stability and preventing tachycardia.
- *Right ventricular dysfunction or pulmonary hypertension*: Directs anesthesiologists to avoid increases in pulmonary vascular resistance and to consider pulmonary vasodilators.
- *Diastolic dysfunction*: May necessitate careful fluid management and heart rate control.

9.9.2 Intraoperative Applications

- In cardiac anesthesia, intraoperative TEE is indispensable.
- In high-risk noncardiac surgery, TEE or transthoracic echocardiography may be used for hemodynamic guidance.

9.9.3 Why It Matters for Anesthesiologists

Even when internists conclude that echocardiographic findings do not alter chronic management, anesthesiologists may modify induction strategy, choice of anesthetic drugs, or monitoring intensity based on echo results.

9.10 Additional Imaging and Ancillary Studies

1. *Chest X-ray*
   - Often low yield for internists in stable patients, but anesthesiologists use it to evaluate:
     - Airway deviation (e.g., from goiter and mediastinal mass).
     - Cardiomegaly, pulmonary congestion, or effusions affecting the induction strategy.
     - Presence of indwelling devices (pacemakers, Implantable Cardioverter-Defibrillator (ICDs), and catheters).
2. *Pulmonary function tests*
   - Rarely routine, but helpful before thoracic surgery or in severe COPD/interstitial lung disease (ILD).
   - Inform the feasibility of one-lung ventilation, risk of postoperative respiratory failure, and extubation planning.
3. *Stress testing/myocardial perfusion imaging*
   - More common in internist-driven evaluation.
   - For anesthesiologists, results provide context for intraoperative ischemia monitoring and thresholds for hemodynamic interventions.
4. *Carotid duplex ultrasound*
   - Performed preoperatively in some vascular surgery patients.
   - Informs anesthesiologists about cerebral perfusion risk and blood pressure management goals.
5. *Computed tomography or magnetic resonance imaging of neck/chest*
   - Particularly relevant in patients with known head-and-neck tumors, mediastinal masses, or tracheal stenosis.
   - Helps anesthesiologists anticipate difficult airway management and induction risk (e.g., airway collapse under anesthesia).

9.11 Conclusion

From the anesthesiologist's perspective, perioperative testing is not merely about identifying chronic disease but about anticipating and managing acute perioperative physiology. CBC informs transfusion thresholds and neuraxial safety; CMP highlights risks of arrhythmia, renal or hepatic clearance issues; T&S ensures preparedness for hemorrhage; coagulation studies influence anesthetic technique and transfusion plans; ECG provides essential baselines for intraoperative interpretation; and echocardiography translates into real-time induction and monitoring strategies.

For internists, recognizing this perspective underscores why anesthesiologists may request or emphasize certain tests even when long-term management would remain unchanged. It reflects the anesthesiologist's mandate to safeguard patients through the vulnerable perioperative period, where small details can dictate major outcomes.

Key Takeaways

1. Anesthesiologists view tests dynamically as tools to anticipate acute perioperative physiology rather than long-term disease burden.
2. CBC and coagulation studies inform transfusion readiness and neuraxial safety, while CMP values guide drug dosing and arrhythmia risk.
3. T&S is critical, even for procedures with expected minimal blood loss, due to the potential for so called unexpected major bleeding.
4. ECG and echocardiography provide intraoperative baselines and guide induction, monitoring, and hemodynamic goals.
5. Selective, guideline-based testing remains the standard, but anesthesiologists may prioritize studies that shape intraoperative planning and crisis management.

Suggested Reading

1. Apfelbaum JL, Connis RT, Nickinovich DG, et al. Practice advisory for preanesthesia evaluation: an updated report by the American Society of Anesthesiologists Task Force on Preanesthesia Evaluation. Anesthesiology. 2012;116(3):522–38.
2. Qaseem A, Snow V, Fitterman N, et al. Risk assessment for and strategies to reduce perioperative pulmonary complications. Ann Intern Med. 2006;144(8):575–80.
3. Kertai MD, Bountioukos M, Boersma E, et al. Aortic stenosis: an underestimated risk factor for perioperative complications in noncardiac surgery. Am J Med. 2004;116(1):8–13.
4. Lepage MA, Lecavalier A, Baldini G, et al. Preoperative risk assessment and optimization integrating surgical and anesthetic principles and practices: a national survey for internists. Perioper Med (Lond). 2025;14(1):6.
5. Subramani S, Tewari A. Pre-operative echocardiography: evidence or experience based utilization in non-cardiac surgery? J Anaesthesiol Clin Pharmacol. 2014;30(3):313–5.

Part III

Anesthesia Pharmacology and Principles of Monitoring

Monitoring Techniques in Anesthesia 10

10.1 Introduction

Monitoring is the cornerstone of modern anesthesiology. Safe anesthetic care requires continuous assessment of the patient's physiological state, detection of adverse events, and timely intervention. Advances in monitoring technology have not only reduced anesthesia-related mortality but also improved outcomes across perioperative, intensive care, and procedural settings.

For internists, familiarity with anesthetic monitoring is essential because many patients experience postoperative complications that often reflect intraoperative events (e.g., myocardial injury, delirium, and neuromuscular weakness). Understanding what anesthesiologists monitor and why provides context for perioperative risk discussions and improves collaborative care.

The American Society of Anesthesiologists (ASA) has established minimum monitoring standards, which apply to every anesthetic regardless of setting. Beyond these, anesthesiologists may employ specialized monitoring techniques tailored to patient comorbidities, surgical complexity, and anesthetic plan.

This chapter reviews the major categories of anesthesia monitoring, including standard ASA monitors, invasive and advanced hemodynamic tools, neuromuscular monitoring, depth of anesthesia monitoring, and emerging technologies such as point-of-care ultrasound (POCUS) and transesophageal echocardiography (TEE). For each, we discuss principles, indications, and relevance to perioperative medicine.

10.2 ASA Standard Monitors

10.2.1 Definition and Scope

The ASA mandates that the following be monitored for every patient receiving anesthesia:

A. Mirrakhimov, *Anesthesiology Demystified for the Internist*,
https://doi.org/10.1007/978-3-032-16811-5_10

- *Oxygenation*: Pulse oximetry and inspired oxygen concentration.
  - *Pulse oximetry*: Detects hypoxemia rapidly, essential for all settings, including procedural sedation.
- *Ventilation*: Capnography (end-tidal CO_2), clinical assessment (e.g., fogging on the oxygen delivery mask, chest expansion), and airway pressure monitoring.
  - *Capnography*: Mandatory for intubated patients, strongly recommended for moderate to deep sedation, detects hypoventilation, disconnection, or esophageal intubation.
- *Circulation*: Continuous ECG, blood pressure (non-invasive or invasive), and pulse palpation.
- *Temperature*: For cases where significant changes are anticipated.

10.2.2 Clinical Significance

Standard monitors are responsible for the dramatic decline in anesthesia-related morbidity and mortality. For internists, the perioperative importance is clear: events such as hypoxemia, hypotension, or arrhythmias detected intraoperatively often manifest later as myocardial injury, delirium, or acute kidney injury.

10.3 Hemodynamic Monitoring

Hemodynamic monitoring extends beyond the basics of ECG and blood pressure. Its purpose is to quantify preload, afterload, contractility, and tissue perfusion.

10.3.1 Non-Invasive Hemodynamic Monitoring

- *Non-invasive blood pressure*: Oscillometric cuffs used in most anesthetics; indicated in stable patients undergoing low- or moderate-risk procedures.
- *Advanced non-invasive cardiac output monitors (e.g., bioimpedance and bioreactance)*: Occasionally used in research or select perioperative scenarios.

10.3.2 Invasive Hemodynamic Monitoring

- *Arterial line*: Provides beat-to-beat blood pressure and access for frequent blood sampling. Indicated for high-risk surgeries (e.g., cardiac, major vascular, and neurosurgical), patients with significant cardiovascular disease, or those requiring tight hemodynamic control.
- *Central venous catheter*: Provides central venous pressure measurement and venous access for vasoactive infusions. Indications include major surgery with expected blood loss, administration of caustic medications, or need for central access.

- *Pulmonary artery catheter (PAC)*: Provides pulmonary pressures, cardiac output, and mixed venous oxygen saturation. Indications are limited today but may include severe pulmonary hypertension, complex cardiac surgery, or advanced heart failure.

10.3.3 Clinical Significance

Hemodynamic monitoring guides intraoperative fluid therapy, vasopressor use, and inotrope administration. For internists, it explains why anesthesiologists request detailed information on baseline cardiac function, medication use, and volume status during preoperative consultations.

10.4 Neuromuscular Monitoring

10.4.1 Principles

Neuromuscular blocking agents (NMBAs) are used to facilitate intubation and optimize surgical conditions. Monitoring their effect is essential to ensure the desired level of muscle relaxation and avoid postoperative residual paralysis from inadequate reversal.

10.4.2 Techniques

- *Peripheral nerve stimulators*: Deliver electrical impulses to a motor nerve (commonly ulnar) and assess muscle response.
- *Train-of-four (TOF)*: Four impulses delivered; fade in twitch amplitude indicates residual blockade.
- *Quantitative monitors (e.g., acceleromyography)*: Provide objective quantitative measurement.

10.4.3 Indications

- All patients receiving NMBAs
- Particularly critical in surgeries requiring deep paralysis (e.g., laparoscopic, thoracic, and neurosurgical)
- Important before extubation to ensure adequate reversal

10.4.4 Clinical Significance

Residual neuromuscular blockade is associated with hypoxemia, aspiration, and delayed recovery. Internists often see its consequences as postoperative respiratory complications, which highlight the importance of intraoperative monitoring.

10.5 Depth of Anesthesia Monitoring

10.5.1 Principles

Depth of anesthesia refers to the patient's level of unconsciousness, analgesia, and amnesia. While clinical signs and hemodynamics provide indirect cues, processed EEG monitors offer objective data.

10.5.2 Bispectral Index (BIS)

- Processes EEG signals to yield a score (0–100).
- 40–60 corresponds to adequate general anesthesia for most patients.
- BIS is frequently used in clinical practice, particularly for high-risk patients, total intravenous anesthesia (TIVA), and cases where inhaled agent concentrations are not a reliable surrogate for anesthetic depth.

10.5.3 Indications

- Patients at risk of intraoperative awareness (e.g., trauma, cardiac surgery, obstetric emergencies, and TIVA without volatile anesthetics)
- High-risk elderly patients to minimize the risk of overly deep anesthesia and potential postoperative delirium or cognitive dysfunction

10.5.4 Limitations

- BIS values are influenced by muscle activity, hypothermia, and specific anesthetic agents.
- Importantly, although BIS monitoring is widely adopted, randomized controlled trials have not consistently shown a reduction in the incidence of intraoperative awareness compared with standard end-tidal anesthetic gas monitoring.
- Accordingly, BIS should be viewed as an adjunct to but not a replacement for comprehensive clinical and anesthetic vigilance.

10.5.5 Clinical Significance

Awareness under anesthesia, though rare, can have psychologically devastating consequences. Excessive anesthetic depth, conversely, may contribute to intraoperative hypotension and postoperative delirium. Depth monitoring provides anesthesiologists with additional data to titrate anesthetics precisely, but its limitations must be recognized.

10.5.6 Urine Output Monitoring

10.5.6.1 Principles and Indications

Intraoperative urine output monitoring, typically achieved via a Foley catheter, provides an indirect assessment of renal perfusion, intravascular volume status, and end-organ function. In the vast majority of situations, it is placed by the circulating operating room nurse. It is commonly placed in:

- Major surgeries with expected fluid shifts or blood loss (e.g., cardiac, abdominal, vascular)
- Prolonged procedures
- Cases where intraoperative diuresis (e.g., mannitol use in neurosurgery) requires quantification

10.5.6.2 Risks and Considerations

Potential risks include urinary tract infection, urethral trauma, hematuria, and discomfort. Difficult catheter placement may occur in patients with urologic pathology, prior instrumentation, or anatomical variations; in such instances, assistance may be requested from the urology team.

10.5.6.3 Clinical Significance

Although not universally required, urine output monitoring can serve as an early warning sign of inadequate perfusion or impending renal injury.

10.6 POCUS and TEE

10.6.1 POCUS

POCUS has revolutionized perioperative monitoring by providing real-time, bedside visualization of anatomy and physiology.

- *Airway*: Confirmation of endotracheal intubation, assessment of airway anatomy
- *Lung*: Diagnosis of pneumothorax, pulmonary edema, pleural effusion, and atelectasis

- *Cardiac*: Focused assessment of ventricular function, pericardial effusion, and volume status
- *Vascular*: Guidance for central venous and arterial catheter placement

Indications:

- Rapid assessment of unexplained hemodynamic instability
- Workup of dyspnea and chest pain
- Trauma and critical illness
- Guidance for line placement and regional blocks

10.6.2 Trans Esophageal Echocardiography (TEE)

TEE is the gold standard for intraoperative cardiac imaging.

- *Indications*:
  - Cardiac surgery (valve, coronary artery bypass graft surgery (CABG), and congenital)
  - Aortic surgery
  - Major non-cardiac surgery (e.g., lung transplantation and liver transplantation)
  - Hemodynamically unstable patients where transthoracic echocardiography (TTE) is inadequate (e.g., poor windows) as part of rescue TEE
  - Monitoring for emboli or air in high-risk procedures (e.g., craniotomy)
- *Contraindications*:
  - Esophageal stricture
  - Esophageal trauma (e.g., perforation)
  - Active upper gastrointestinal bleeding
  - Esophageal tumor
  - Esophagectomy
  - History of radiation to neck/chest (relative)
  - Barrett's esophagus (relative)
  - Hiatal hernia (relative)
  - Dysphagia (relative)
  - Restriction in cervical mobility (relative)
  - Varices (relative)
  - Esophagitis (relative)
  - Coagulopathy (relative)
- *Capabilities*:
  - Real-time assessment of ventricular filling and contractility
  - Valvular structure and function
  - Guidance during valve repair/replacement and congenital repairs
  - Detection of wall motion abnormalities

10.6.3 Clinical Significance

POCUS and TEE extend monitoring beyond numbers to direct visualization of pathology. For internists, these tools exemplify the growing overlap between anesthesiology and internal medicine, particularly critical care and cardiology.

10.7 Conclusion

Monitoring is inseparable from the practice of safe anesthesia. From the universally applied ASA standard monitors to advanced modalities such as TEE and POCUS, each tool has specific indications that tailor anesthetic care to the patient's risks and the surgical demands.

For internists, understanding these monitoring strategies clarifies how anesthesiologists anticipate, detect, and respond to perioperative events. More importantly, it highlights how intraoperative data inform postoperative outcomes, strengthening collaboration between specialties in the shared goal of optimizing patient safety.

Not all monitors have been shown to improve hard outcomes; for example, BIS monitoring, while widely used, has not conclusively been shown to lower awareness risk compared with standard practice. This underscores that monitoring complements but never replaces clinical judgment and vigilance, the hallmarks of anesthesiology.

Key Takeaways

1. ASA standards—oxygenation, ventilation, circulation, and temperature—apply to all anesthetics as the universal minimum.
2. Invasive hemodynamic monitors guide fluid, vasopressor, and resuscitation strategies in high-risk patients and complex surgeries.
3. Neuromuscular monitoring is critical to ensure safe paralysis and reversal, preventing residual weakness and aspiration.
4. Depth of anesthesia monitors like BIS are useful adjuncts but cannot substitute for comprehensive anesthetic vigilance.
5. POCUS and TEE expand monitoring into real-time imaging of physiology, strengthening perioperative care and internist–anesthesiologist collaboration.

Suggested Reading

1. American Society of Anesthesiologists. Standards for basic anesthetic monitoring. ASA House of Delegates; 2020. https://www.asahq.org/standards-and-practice-parameters/standards-for-basic-anesthetic-monitoring.
2. Deng Y, Cruz Navarro J, Markan S. Advances in anesthesia monitoring. Oral Maxillofac Surg Clin North Am. 2019;31(4):611–9.
3. Naguib M, Brull SJ, Kopman AF, et al. Consensus statement on perioperative use of neuromuscular monitoring. Anesth Analg. 2018;127(1):71–80.

4. Punjasawadwong Y, Phongchiewboon A, Bunchungmongkol N. Bispectral index for improving anesthetic delivery and postoperative recovery. Cochrane Database Syst Rev. 2014;(6):CD003843.
5. Li L, Yong RJ, Kaye AD, et al. Perioperative Point of Care Ultrasound (POCUS) for anesthesiologists: an overview. Curr Pain Headache Rep. 2020;24(5):20.
6. Rong LQ, Shore-Lesserson L, Belani K, et al. Considerations of intraoperative transesophageal echocardiography during adult cardiac surgery: a scientific statement from the American Heart Association. Circulation. 2025;152(2):129–45.
7. Efrimescu CI, Moorthy A, Griffin M. Rescue transesophageal echocardiography: a narrative review of current knowledge and practice. J Cardiothorac Vasc Anesth. 2023;37(4):584–600.
8. Fayad A, Shillcutt SK. Perioperative transesophageal echocardiography for non-cardiac surgery. Can J Anaesth. 2017;65(4):381–98.
9. Hahn RT, Abraham T, Adams MS, et al. Guidelines for performing a comprehensive transesophageal echocardiographic examination: recommendations from the American Society of Echocardiography and the Society of Cardiovascular Anesthesiologists. J Am Soc Echocardiogr. 2013;26(9):921–64.

Core Anesthetic Agents: Intravenous Agents, Inhalational Anesthetics, and Neuromuscular Blockers

11

11.1 Introduction

Modern anesthesia relies on a relatively short but powerful list of pharmacologic agents that permit the controlled induction and maintenance of unconsciousness, amnesia, analgesia, and immobility. Anesthesiologists deploy these drugs with precision, tailoring them to the patient's comorbidities, surgical demands, and anticipated physiologic perturbations.

A practical distinction is that in most adult anesthetics, intravenous (IV) agents are used for induction, providing rapid loss of consciousness and airway control, whereas inhalational agents are used primarily for maintenance, allowing steady depth of anesthesia and rapid titration. Exceptions exist, such as inhalational induction in pediatrics (many pediatric patients will not tolerate the placement of an IV catheter while awake), but this principle guides most adult anesthesia practice.

This chapter reviews core anesthetic agents from the anesthesiologist's perspective: pharmacological class, mechanism of action, pharmacokinetics (onset, duration after single dose, and infusion), pharmacodynamics, clinical roles, side effects, contraindications, and high-yield drug interactions.

11.2 Anesthetic Agents

11.2.1 Propofol

- *Class:* Alkylphenol hypnotic.
- *Mechanism:* Potentiates Gamma-aminobutyric acid type A (GABA-A) receptor activity, increasing chloride conductance and neuronal hyperpolarization, leading to hypnosis.

11.2.1.1 Pharmacokinetics

- *Onset:* 30–45 s after IV bolus.

A. Mirrakhimov, *Anesthesiology Demystified for the Internist*,
https://doi.org/10.1007/978-3-032-16811-5_11

- *Duration single dose:* 5–10 min.
- *Infusion:* Context-sensitive half-time (the time for plasma drug concentration to decrease by 50% after stopping an infusion, dependent on infusion duration) remains short, even with prolonged infusion.

11.2.1.2 Pharmacodynamics and Role

- Produces hypnosis, amnesia, and antiemetic effects, but lacks intrinsic analgesia.
- Causes vasodilation and mild myocardial depression → hypotension.
- *Role in anesthesia:* Commonly used for the induction of general anesthesia. Also used for sedation in endoscopy, procedural settings, and intensive care units (ICUs).

11.2.1.3 Side Effects/Contraindications

- Hypotension, apnea, pain on injection.
- Rare: Propofol infusion syndrome (with prolonged high-dose infusion).
- Avoid in severe hemodynamic instability unless vasopressors are available.

11.2.2 Etomidate

- *Class:* Imidazole derivative hypnotic.
- *Mechanism:* Potentiates GABA-A receptor activity, enhancing chloride flux and neuronal inhibition.

11.2.2.1 Pharmacokinetics

- *Onset:* 30–60 s.
- *Duration (single dose):* 5–10 min (rapid redistribution).
- *Duration (infusion):* Accumulates with prolonged use; recovery is longer than propofol. Continuous infusion of etomidate is not typically employed because of its association with adrenal suppression.

11.2.2.2 Pharmacodynamics and Role

- Provides hypnosis with minimal cardiovascular depression.
- Maintains hemodynamic stability: heart rate and blood pressure remain relatively preserved.
- *Role in anesthesia:* Induction agent of choice for patients with poor cardiac reserve (minimal hemodynamic effects), severe valvular disease, hypovolemia, or major trauma. Also widely used in rapid sequence intubation in critically ill patients.
- No analgesic properties.

11.2.2.3 Side Effects/Contraindications

- Adrenocortical suppression (inhibits 11β-hydroxylase): even a single dose transiently decreases cortisol and aldosterone synthesis. Prolonged infusions are avoided in ICU sedation due to its association with an increased mortality risk.

- Myoclonus and seizure-like movements (reduced with benzodiazepine or opioid pretreatment).
- Pain on injection.
- Nausea and vomiting are more common than with propofol.

11.2.3 Barbiturates (Thiopental and Methohexital)

- *Class:* Barbiturate hypnotics.
- *Mechanism:* Potentiate GABA-A by prolonging chloride channel opening; at high doses can directly activate GABA-A.

11.2.3.1 Pharmacokinetics

- *Onset:* 20–30 s.
- *Duration single dose:* 5–10 min (redistribution).
- *Infusion:* Accumulate in fat → prolonged recovery.

11.2.3.2 Pharmacodynamics and Clinical Role

- Produce profound hypnosis, cerebral metabolic suppression, and anticonvulsant effects.
- Historically used for the induction of general anesthesia; now largely replaced by propofol.

11.2.3.3 Thiopental

- Once widely used, thiopental is no longer available in the United States due to manufacturing and regulatory issues, though it remains in use in some countries. It is still valued abroad for neuroprotection (e.g., during refractory intracranial hypertension or neurosurgical cases).

11.2.3.4 Methohexital

- Methohexital is the agent of choice for electroconvulsive therapy (ECT) because it provides a rapid onset and very short duration of action, allowing quick recovery between treatments. Critically, methohexital has pro-convulsant properties, lowering seizure threshold and supporting robust therapeutic seizures, which is important for ECT. In contrast, propofol often shortens seizure duration, potentially diminishing ECT efficacy.
- Methohexital thus balances reliable induction, rapid emergence, and seizure augmentation, making it well-suited to ECT.

11.2.3.5 Side Effects/Contraindications

- Hypotension, respiratory depression.
- Porphyrinogenic → contraindicated in acute intermittent porphyria.

11.2.4 Benzodiazepines (Midazolam, Lorazepam, and Diazepam)

- *Class:* Benzodiazepines.
- *Mechanism:* Bind to the benzodiazepine site on GABA-A, enhancing the frequency of chloride channel opening in the presence of GABA.

11.2.4.1 Pharmacokinetics

- *Midazolam:* Onset 2–3 min; duration after a single dose 15–30 min. Infusion → prolonged recovery.
- *Lorazepam:* Onset 5–10 min; duration 6–8 h (slower redistribution, higher receptor affinity). Infusion → marked accumulation.
- *Diazepam:* Onset 2–3 min; duration 1–2 h, single dose. Elimination half-life >20 h; active metabolites prolong the effect.

11.2.4.2 Pharmacodynamics

- All benzodiazepines provide anxiolysis, amnesia, hypnosis, minor muscle relaxation (insufficient for surgical immobility), and anticonvulsant effects.
- *Midazolam:* Rapid onset, short acting → most common for premedication and procedural sedation.
- *Lorazepam:* Strong binding and slower redistribution → potent amnestic and anticonvulsant. Often used in ICU sedation and seizure management, but not favored for OR due to long recovery.
- *Diazepam:* Long-acting with robust anticonvulsant and anxiolytic effects; less used intraoperatively due to slow recovery, but relevant in sedation, seizure control, and muscle spasm management.

11.2.4.3 Role in Anesthesia

- Used mainly for premedication, anxiolysis, and amnesia.
- Rarely used as sole induction agents due to slow onset and prolonged recovery (except historically or in special settings).

11.2.4.4 Side Effects/Contraindications

- Respiratory depression, synergistic with opioids and other sedatives.
- Hypotension in frail patients.
- Delirium in elderly patients.
- Avoid in severe respiratory failure without airway support.

Antagonist: Flumazenil—short acting, may precipitate seizures in chronic users. Of note, the duration of action of flumazenil is shorter than that of most benzodiazepines; therefore, if used to reverse benzodiazepine overdose, the risk of re-sedation must be recognized and patients should be closely monitored.

11.2.5 Ketamine

- *Class:* Phencyclidine derivative.
- *Mechanism:* N-Methyl-D-Aspartate (NMDA) receptor antagonist; also modulates opioid, muscarinic, and monoaminergic receptors.

11.2.5.1 Pharmacokinetics

- *Onset:* 30–60 s IV; 2–4 min IM.
- *Duration after a single dose:* 10–20 min.
- *Duration infusion:* Accumulates with prolonged infusion; emergence is expected within 30–60 min after cessation.

11.2.5.2 Pharmacodynamics and Role

- Produces dissociative anesthesia: profound analgesia, amnesia, catalepsy, while often preserving airway reflexes and spontaneous ventilation.
- Sympathomimetic: ↑ heart rate (HR), blood pressure (BP), and Cardiac output (CO). However, ketamine possesses direct negative inotropic properties, which may explain the occasional occurrence of hypotension in patients with depleted catecholamine stores, such as those experiencing prolonged shock prior to ketamine administration.
- *Role in anesthesia:* Valuable in trauma, hypovolemia, or unstable patients; procedural sedation; patients with reactive airways (bronchodilator). Also used in sub-anesthetic doses for analgesia in multimodal regimens.

11.2.5.3 Side Effects/Contraindications

- Emergence reactions (e.g., hallucinations and nightmares).
- Increased salivation, nausea, and vomiting.
- Increases ICP/IOP → caution in certain neurosurgical/ophthalmic cases.

11.3 Inhalational Anesthetic Agents

11.3.1 General Properties

- *Agents:* Isoflurane, sevoflurane, desflurane, and nitrous oxide. Halothane is no longer used in the United States and is primarily of historical interest because of its association with halothane hepatitis. However, it remains in use in some developing countries due to its low cost and availability.
- *Mechanism:* Likely involves GABA-A, glycine, NMDA, and K+ channel modulation.

11.3.1.1 Role in Anesthesia

- In adults, inhalational agents are primarily used for maintenance following IV induction.
- In children, sevoflurane is often used for inhalational induction due to its non-pungency and smooth uptake.

11.3.1.2 Pharmacokinetics

- Determined by blood-gas solubility.
- *Sevoflurane:* Low solubility, rapid onset and emergence; widely used.
- *Desflurane:* Very low solubility → fastest emergence; pungent, high risk of airway irritation.
- *Isoflurane:* Higher solubility, slower uptake, and longer emergence than sevoflurane.
- *Nitrous oxide:* Minimal hypnotic potency, modest analgesic; used as an adjunct anesthetic (e.g., commonly used in dental practices and may be used in labor analgesia).

11.4 Minimum Alveolar Concentration

The minimum alveolar concentration (MAC) is the standard measure of anesthetic potency for volatile anesthetics. It is defined as the alveolar concentration of an agent at one atmosphere of pressure that prevents movement in 50% of patients exposed to surgical incision.

Several clinically important derivatives of MAC are recognized:

- *MACawake*: The concentration at which 50% of patients will respond to verbal command, typically 0.3–0.5 MAC.
- *MACaware*: The concentration preventing consciousness and awareness in 50% of patients, usually 0.5–0.7 MAC.
- *MACBAR (Block Autonomic Response)*: The concentration preventing adrenergic/autonomic responses (e.g., tachycardia and hypertension) to surgical stimuli in 50% of patients, typically 1.5–2.0 MAC.

MAC Modifiers MAC decreases with advanced age, hypothermia, hypotension, pregnancy, and CNS depressants (opioids, benzodiazepines, and dexmedetomidine), and increases with young age, hyperthermia, chronic alcohol, or stimulant use.

Modern Relevance While MAC is a population-based concept, modern anesthesia workstations enhance its clinical utility by calculating the patient's age-adjusted MAC in real time, based on exhaled volatile anesthetic concentrations (see Fig. 11.1). This provides anesthesiologists with a continuous estimate of anesthetic depth tailored to the individual, although it must still be interpreted alongside physiological parameters and, when applicable, processed Electroencephalogram (EEG) or neuromonitoring.

Clinical Takeaway MAC standardizes anesthetic potency and guides volatile dosing, but individual requirements vary. It should be used as a reference point integrated with patient-specific factors and adjunct monitoring tools, not as an absolute target.

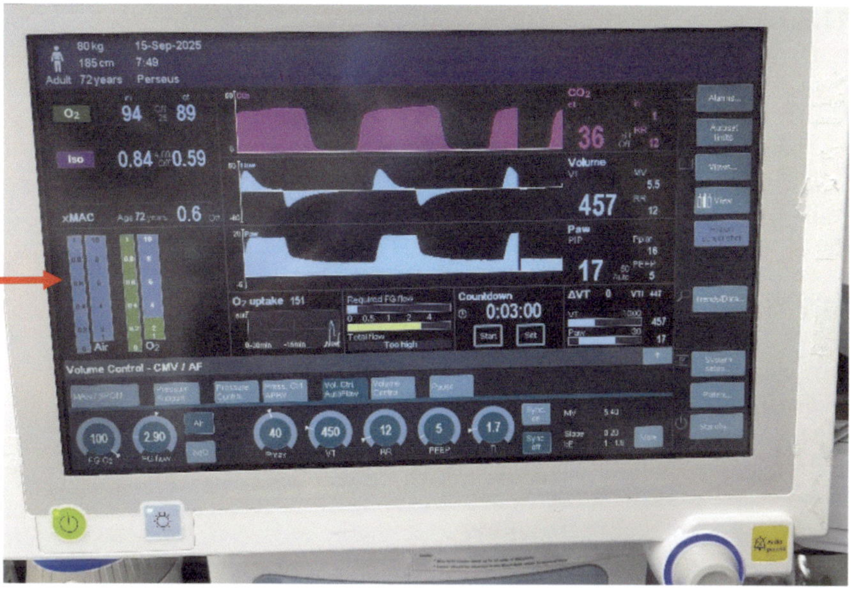

Fig. 11.1 MAC value automatically calculated for the patient (red arrow)

11.4.1 Side Effects/Contraindications

- Hypotension from vasodilation and less from myocardial depression.
- Dose-dependent respiratory depression.
- Malignant hyperthermia trigger (all except nitrous oxide). Volatile anesthetics must be avoided for patients at risk for malignant hyperthermia.
- Nitrous oxide is contraindicated in pneumothorax, bowel obstruction, and intracranial air (can increase the size and volume).

11.5 Neuromuscular Blocking Agents

11.5.1 Depolarizing: Succinylcholine

- *Mechanism:* Nicotinic receptor agonist → depolarization → flaccid paralysis.
- *Onset:* 30–60 s.
- *Duration single dose:* 5–10 min (in most patients; however, the duration may extend to several hours in those with pseudocholinesterase deficiency, a rare condition.)
- *Role:* Gold standard for rapid sequence induction (RSI) due to rapid onset/offset.
- *Reversal agent:* None is available. Neuromuscular function is restored through the metabolism and redistribution of succinylcholine.

11.5.1.1 Side Effects/Contraindications

- Hyperkalemia: This can be pronounced in patients with burns or neuromuscular disorders, potentially precipitating severe cardiac arrhythmias or even cardiac arrest.
- Malignant hyperthermia trigger (must be avoided in patients with a history of malignant hyperthermia).
- Bradycardia in pediatrics.

11.5.2 Non-depolarizing Agents

- *Aminosteroids:* Rocuronium and vecuronium.
- *Benzylisoquinoliniums:* Atracurium and cisatracurium.

Mechanism: Competitive antagonists at nicotinic acetylcholine receptors.

11.5.2.1 Pharmacokinetics/Role

- *Rocuronium:* Onset 60–90 s (at RSI dose); duration 30–60 min. RSI alternative to succinylcholine.
- *Vecuronium:* Onset 2–3 min, duration 30–40 min.
- *Cisatracurium:* Onset 2–3 min, duration 30–40 min; Hofmann elimination → organ-independent clearance, preferred in renal/hepatic failure.

11.5.2.2 Reversal

- *Neostigmine* (acetylcholinesterase inhibitor) for all non-depolarizing neuromuscular blockers. Neostigmine is suboptimal for reversal of a deep neuromuscular blockade. Patients in this state should remain mechanically ventilated and sedated until sufficient spontaneous recovery of neuromuscular function has occurred (if sugammadex is not available) to permit the safe and effective use of neostigmine.
- *Sugammadex*: Encapsulates rocuronium/vecuronium, allowing rapid, complete reversal. Ineffective for atracurium and cisatracurium.

11.5.2.3 Side Effects/Interactions

- Residual weakness if not reversed.
- Histamine release (atracurium).
- Potentiated by volatile anesthetics, aminoglycosides, and magnesium.

11.6 Conclusion

Core anesthetic agents such as IV sedatives, inhalational agents, and neuromuscular blockers form the pharmacologic backbone of modern anesthesiology. IV drugs such as propofol remain the mainstay for induction, while inhalational agents dominate maintenance in adults. Barbiturates are largely historical, but methohexital retains a vital role in ECT. Benzodiazepines provide anxiolysis and amnesia, with pharmacodynamic differences among midazolam, lorazepam, and diazepam. Ketamine offers unique dissociative anesthesia, especially in unstable patients. Neuromuscular blockers allow airway control and surgical immobility, with succinylcholine irreplaceable for RSI and non-depolarizers central to routine practice.

Understanding their pharmacology and context-specific applications enables internists to better appreciate anesthesiologists' decision-making and anticipate perioperative physiology.

Key Takeaways

1. Division of labor: IV agents usually for induction; volatiles for maintenance (pediatric exception: inhalational induction).
2. Hemodynamics matter: Propofol lowers BP; etomidate preserves stability but suppresses adrenal steroidogenesis; ketamine supports BP/bronchial tone in most patients.
3. Volatile essentials: Solubility dictates speed; all volatiles (not N_2O) are MH triggers.
4. Paralysis and reversal: Use objective neuromuscular monitoring and appropriate reversal.
5. High-yield cautions: Propofol infusion syndrome, etomidate adrenal suppression, ketamine emergence reactions, and N_2O in closed gas spaces.

Suggested Reading

1. Khan KS, Hayes I, Buggy DJ. Pharmacology of anaesthetic agents I: intravenous anaesthetic agents. Contin Educ Anaesth Crit Care Pain. 2014;14(3):100–5.
2. Khan KS, Hayes I, Buggy DJ. Pharmacology of anaesthetic agents II: inhalation anaesthetic agents. Contin Educ Anaesth Crit Care Pain. 2014;14(3):106–11.
3. Naguib M, Brull SJ, Kopman AF, et al. Consensus statement on perioperative use of neuromuscular monitoring. Anesth Analg. 2018;127(1):71–80.
4. Brown EN, Pavone KJ, Naranjo M. Multimodal general anesthesia: theory and practice. Anesth Analg. 2018;127(5):1246–58.
5. Rodney G, Raju P, Brull SJ. Neuromuscular block management: evidence-based principles and practice. BJA Educ. 2024;24(1):13–22.
6. Welhengama C, Hall A, Hunter JM. Neuromuscular blocking drugs in the critically ill. BJA Educ. 2021;21(7):258–63.

12 Pharmacological Adjuncts and Special Medications: Opioids, Dexmedetomidine, and Local Anesthetics

12.1 Introduction

While hypnotic agents induce unconsciousness and neuromuscular blockers provide immobility, adjunctive medications are essential to create a balanced anesthetic state. These agents allow anesthesiologists to optimize analgesia, sedation, hemodynamic stability, and recovery, while reducing reliance on volatile anesthetics.

This chapter focuses on opioids, dexmedetomidine, and local anesthetics—three categories of agents that shape modern perioperative care.

12.2 Opioids

12.2.1 Opioid Receptors: A Brief Overview

Opioids act on G-protein-coupled receptors located in the central and peripheral nervous system. Their effects are receptor subtype-specific:

- *μ (Mu) receptors*,
  - Analgesia (supraspinal and spinal).
  - Respiratory depression.
  - Euphoria, dependence.
  - Miosis.
  - Reduced gastrointestinal motility and constipation.
  - Pruritus and urinary retention.
- *κ (Kappa) receptors*,
  - Analgesia (primarily spinal).
  - Sedation.
  - Dysphoria and hallucinations.
  - Diuresis.

A. Mirrakhimov, *Anesthesiology Demystified for the Internist*,
https://doi.org/10.1007/978-3-032-16811-5_12

- *δ (Delta) receptors,*
  - Analgesia (spinal and peripheral).
  - May modulate emotional response to pain.
  - Less clinically exploited but contribute to tolerance mechanisms.

Most opioids used in anesthesia practice are μ-agonists. Differences in potency, onset, and context-sensitive half-time shape their role in perioperative care.

12.2.2 Morphine

- *Mechanism:* μ-agonist.
- *Onset:* 5–10 min intravenous (IV).
- *Duration of action (bolus):* 3–4 hours.
- *Duration of action (infusion):* Accumulates with repeated dosing (especially in patients with renal and liver dysfunction).
- *Role:* Moderate to severe pain; intra- and postoperative analgesia. Not favored as an adjunct to the induction of general anesthesia (compared to fentanyl, sufentanil, or remifentanil) due to a slower onset.
- *Side effects:* Histamine release (hypotension, pruritus), respiratory depression, and nausea.
- *Contraindications:* Renal failure (active metabolite accumulation) and severe respiratory depression.

12.2.3 Fentanyl

- *Mechanism:* Potent μ-agonist.
- *Onset:* 1–2 min IV.
- *Duration of action (bolus):* 30–60 minutes
- *Duration of action (infusion):* Context-sensitive half-time lengthens with prolonged infusion.
- *Role:* Commonly used opioid intraoperatively; blunts sympathetic response to intubation and surgical stimulation.
- *Side effects:* Respiratory depression, bradycardia, and chest wall rigidity with rapid/high doses. Potential risk of serotonin syndrome when combined with other agents (e.g., Selective Serotonin Reuptake Inhibitor (SSRI), ondansetron, etc.).

12.2.4 Hydromorphone

- *Mechanism:* μ-agonist.
- *Onset:* ~5 minutes IV.

- *Duration of action (bolus):* 3–4 hours.
- *Role:* Provides longer-lasting analgesia than fentanyl. Often chosen for postoperative analgesia.
- *Side effects:* Less histamine release than morphine. It accumulates in renal/hepatic impairment but overall lower risk than morphine. Its main metabolite, hydromorphone-3-glucuronide (H3G), lacks analgesic activity, but neurotoxicity can still occur.

12.2.5 Sufentanil

- *Mechanism:* Very potent μ-agonist.
- *Onset:* 1–2 minutes IV.
- *Duration of action (bolus):* 30–45 minutes.
- *Duration of action (infusion):* More favorable context-sensitive half-time compared to fentanyl.
- *Role:* Cardiac and major surgery, where potency and stable kinetics are beneficial.
- *Side effects:* Severe respiratory depression and chest wall rigidity (like fentanyl).

12.2.6 Remifentanil

- *Mechanism:* Potent μ-agonist.
- *Onset:* ~1 minute IV.
- *Duration (bolus):* 5–10 minutes.
- *Duration (infusion):* Context-sensitive half-time independent of infusion duration (unique metabolism by nonspecific esterases).
- *Role:* Ideal for cases requiring intense analgesia with rapid offset (neurosurgery, airway surgery, and cardiac procedures). Not used for postoperative analgesia.
- *Side effects:* Bradycardia, hypotension, and rapid hyperalgesia after discontinuation.

12.2.7 Methadone (IV)

- *Mechanism:* μ-agonist, N-methyl-D-aspartate (NMDA) receptor antagonist, and serotonin/norepinephrine reuptake inhibitor.
- *Onset:* ~10 minutes IV.
- *Duration of action (bolus):* 4–6 hours analgesia; elimination half-life ~24 hours.
- *Role:* Provides long-acting intra- and postoperative analgesia, reduces opioid tolerance and hyperalgesia.
- *Side effects:* Respiratory depression; QT prolongation and torsades risk.
- *Contraindications:* Prolonged baseline QTc, concurrent QT-prolonging medications. Risk of serotonin syndrome, especially when combined with other agents (e.g., SSRI, ondansetron, linezolid, etc.)

12.3 Dexmedetomidine

- *Class:* Highly selective α2-adrenergic agonist.
- *Mechanism:* Acts in the locus coeruleus (sedation) and dorsal horn (analgesia). Produces "cooperative sedation" resembling natural sleep.

12.3.1 Pharmacokinetics

- *Onset:* 5–10 minutes IV after bolus. The onset of action may be delayed if a loading (bolus) dose is not administered and only a continuous infusion is initiated (~30 minutes).
- *Duration of action (bolus):* 30–60 minutes.
- *Duration (infusion):* Context-sensitive half-time ~ 4 minute, but clinical recovery gets slower with prolonged infusion.

12.3.2 Role in Anesthesia

- Adjunct to reduce volatile and opioid requirements.
- Facilitates awake fiberoptic intubation.
- Intensive care unit (ICU) sedation: associated with less delirium compared to benzodiazepines.
- Perioperative analgesic adjunct.

12.3.3 Side Effects/Contraindications

- Bradycardia.
- Hypertension with rapid bolus (peripheral α2B activation on vascular smooth muscle leading to vasoconstriction).
- Hypotension (common with prolonged infusion).
- Contraindicated in advanced AV block without pacing capabilities.
- Provides poor and unreliable amnesia and weak sedation, insufficient to produce general anesthesia at standard doses; therefore, it should not be used as a sole agent when deep sedation is required (e.g., in patients receiving neuromuscular blockade).

12.4 Local Anesthetics

12.4.1 Mechanism and Classification

Local anesthetics block voltage-gated sodium channels, inhibiting action potential propagation.

- *Esters* (procaine, chloroprocaine, and tetracaine): hydrolyzed by plasma cholinesterases; shorter duration, higher allergy potential.
- *Amides* (lidocaine, mepivacaine, ropivacaine, and bupivacaine): metabolized hepatically; longer-acting, lower allergy risk.

12.4.2 IV Lidocaine as an Adjunct

- *Role:* Intraoperative infusion decreases pain, opioid use, and ileus; blunts airway reflexes during induction and intubation. May reduce the risk of ventricular arrhythmias under anesthesia. Lidocaine is the only local anesthetic commonly administered IV; other local anesthetics are typically employed for local tissue infiltration, peripheral nerve blocks, or neuraxial anesthesia.
- *Onset:* Within 1 minute after IV administration.
- *Duration:* Rapid clearance; effects dissipate within 20–30 minutes after infusion ends.
- *Side effects:* Central nervous system (CNS) toxicity (tinnitus and seizures); cardiac toxicity at high concentrations.

12.4.3 Commonly Used Agents (for Regional and Neuraxial Anesthesia)

12.4.3.1 Lidocaine

- *Onset:* 2–3 minutes.
- *Duration (infiltration):* 1–2 hours; 2–4 hours when combined with epinephrine (reduced vascular uptake).
- *Role:* Local infiltration, nerve blocks, epidural use when a quick onset is needed, IV adjunct.
- *Side effects:* risk of local anesthetic systemic toxicity (LAST).

12.4.3.2 Mepivacaine

- *Onset:* 2–4 minutes.
- *Duration:* 2–3 hours.
- *Role:* Peripheral blocks, epidurals. Avoid IV administration.
- *Side effects:* Similar to lidocaine, less vasodilation.

12.4.3.3 Ropivacaine

- *Onset:* 10–15 minutes.
- *Duration:* 4–6 hours.
- *Role:* Peripheral and neuraxial blocks; less cardiotoxic than bupivacaine. Avoid IV administration.
- *Side effects:* CNS excitation; rare severe cardiac toxicity.

12.4.3.4 Bupivacaine

- *Onset:* 5–10 minutes.
- *Duration:* 4–8 hours (long-acting).
- *Role:* Spinal, epidural, and peripheral nerve blocks.
- *Side effects: Highest cardiotoxic risk*—ventricular arrhythmias, cardiac arrest. Avoid IV administration.

12.4.4 Toxicity and Management

- *LAST (see Chap. 27 for more information):* CNS symptoms (perioral numbness and seizures) progressing to cardiovascular collapse.
- *Treatment:* Airway support, benzodiazepines for seizures, and 20% intralipid therapy.
- *Contraindications:* True allergy (rare); relative caution in severe hepatic dysfunction for amides.

12.5 Conclusion

Adjunctive agents are indispensable to balanced anesthesia. Opioids, acting mainly on μ receptors, remain the foundation of perioperative analgesia, with agents tailored to procedure length and recovery needs. Dexmedetomidine offers sedation and analgesia without respiratory depression but requires vigilance for bradycardia and hypotension. Local anesthetics, systemically or regionally, are essential to multimodal analgesia and regional techniques, though their toxicities mandate respect and readiness with lipid rescue therapy.

For internists, appreciating these adjuncts clarifies anesthesiologists' perioperative planning, monitoring requests, and complication management.

Key Takeaways

1. Opioids remain central to perioperative analgesia, with agent selection guided by potency, duration, and surgical context.
2. Dexmedetomidine provides cooperative sedation with opioid-sparing benefits but carries risks of bradycardia and blood pressure fluctuations.
3. Local anesthetics enable regional and systemic analgesia, improving recovery and reducing opioid requirements.
4. LAST is a rare but life-threatening complication, requiring immediate lipid rescue therapy.
5. Balanced anesthesia with adjuncts minimizes complications, optimizes recovery, and underlines the importance of multimodal analgesia.

Suggested Reading

1. Egan TD. Are opioids indispensable for general anaesthesia? Br J Anaesth. 2019;122(6):e127–35.
2. Adams TJ, Aljohani DM, Forget P. Perioperative opioids: a narrative review contextualising new avenues to improve prescribing. Br J Anaesth. 2023;130(6):709–18.
3. Kharasch ED. Intraoperative methadone and postoperative anesthesia care unit outcomes: a retrospective cohort analysis. Anesthesiology. 2024;141(2):408–10.
4. Lee S. Dexmedetomidine: present and future directions. Korean J Anesthesiol. 2019;72(4):323–30.
5. Kranke P, Jokinen J, Pace NL, et al. Continuous intravenous lidocaine for postoperative pain. Cochrane Database Syst Rev. 2015;(7):CD009642.
6. Taylor A, McLeod G. Basic pharmacology of local anaesthetics. BJA Educ. 2020;20(2):34–41.
7. Becker DE, Reed KL. Local anesthetics: review of pharmacological considerations. Anesth Prog. 2012;59(2):90–101.

Part IV

Types of Anesthesia and Surgical Positioning

Monitored Anesthesia Care 13

13.1 Introduction

Monitored Anesthesia Care (MAC) is a widely utilized anesthetic technique that integrates vigilant physiologic monitoring, carefully titrated pharmacologic sedation, and preparedness to convert to general anesthesia when clinically indicated. Although often perceived as a "lighter" or "simpler" alternative to general anesthesia, MAC requires equal, if not greater, vigilance and expertise from the anesthesia professional. The anesthesiologist must simultaneously ensure patient comfort, hemodynamic stability, and safety, while maintaining a constant state of readiness to manage airway compromise or transition to deeper anesthetic levels if necessary.

Internists frequently encounter patients undergoing procedures under MAC, ranging from endoscopy and interventional radiology to ophthalmic and minor vascular surgery. Understanding MAC's defining features, its distinction from sedation alone, and the clinical decision-making that guides its use is essential for collaborative perioperative care.

13.2 Core Features of MAC

According to the American Society of Anesthesiologists (ASA), MAC is a distinct anesthetic service and not merely "sedation." Its defining features include:

- Comprehensive monitoring equivalent to that used in general anesthesia (continuous pulse oximetry, ECG, blood pressure, and increasingly capnography).
- Titrated administration of sedatives, analgesics, and/or anxiolytics to provide patient comfort while usually preserving spontaneous ventilation and hemodynamic stability.

A. Mirrakhimov, *Anesthesiology Demystified for the Internist*,
https://doi.org/10.1007/978-3-032-16811-5_13

- Immediate availability of advanced airway management and resuscitation skills and equipment.
- Preparedness to convert to general anesthesia at any time if patient safety or procedural conditions require.

Thus, MAC is best understood as anesthesia care with sedation and monitoring, rather than "sedation alone."

13.3 MAC Versus Sedation

Sedation exists along a continuum, from light anxiolysis to deep sedation. In some contexts, sedation may be administered by non-anesthesiologists, but MAC always involves an anesthesia professional capable of transitioning to general anesthesia.

13.3.1 Key Distinctions

- Sedation alone prioritizes comfort but may lack immediate resources for airway rescue or hemodynamic support.
- MAC ensures anesthesiologist-level vigilance, ASA-standard monitoring, and immediate readiness for advanced interventions.

13.4 Levels of Sedation and Anesthesia

The ASA defines four levels of sedation along the sedation–anesthesia continuum. The levels of sedation and their associated clinical characteristics are summarized in Table 13.1.

Table 13.1 Levels of sedation

Feature	Minimal sedation (Anxiolysis)	Moderate sedation ("Conscious sedation")	Deep sedation	General anesthesia
Responsiveness	Normal response to verbal stimuli	Purposeful response to verbal/tactile stimuli	Purposeful response after repeated or painful stimuli	Unarousable even with painful stimuli
Airway	Unaffected	No intervention required	Intervention may be required	Intervention often required
Spontaneous ventilation	Unaffected	Adequate	May be inadequate	Frequently inadequate and requires support
Cardiovascular function	Unaffected	Usually maintained	Usually maintained	May be impaired

MAC may encompass any level of sedation, even general anesthesia if required by the clinical situation. What distinguishes MAC is the continuous presence of an anesthesia provider with full rescue capability.

13.5 Pharmacology in MAC

Commonly used medications during MAC include (see Chaps. 11 and 12 for more information):

- *Midazolam* (anxiolysis, amnesia).
- *Propofol* (titrated hypnosis, rapid recovery).
- *Dexmedetomidine* (cooperative sedation, minimal respiratory depression).
- *Opioids* (fentanyl, remifentanil for analgesia).
- *Ketamine* (analgesia, amnesia, preserved reflexes in selected patients).
- *Adjuncts* (IV lidocaine, regional blocks) to minimize systemic sedative and opioid needs.

The choice and titration of drugs depend on patient comorbidities, procedure type, and the need to maintain airway safety.

13.6 Patient Selection for MAC

13.6.1 Appropriate Candidates

- Low-to-moderate anesthetic risk (ASA I–III).
- Patients with stable comorbidities who can tolerate moderate or deeper levels of sedation.
- Cooperative individuals able to remain relatively still and responsive.

13.6.2 Poor Candidates for MAC

Certain patient factors make MAC less suitable because they increase the likelihood of sedation failure or unplanned conversion to general anesthesia under suboptimal circumstances:

- *Severe anxiety or psychiatric illness* (patients should be willing to accept a chance of procedure-related memory and awareness).
- *Expected procedure-related pain* and stimulation should be matched to the patient's pain tolerance. Procedures that are highly painful or intensely stimulating are generally not suitable for MAC.
- *Cognitive impairment or dementia*, which limits cooperation or the ability to follow instructions.

- *Language barriers* without reliable interpreter support complicate the assessment of responsiveness.
- *Severe obstructive sleep apnea or morbid obesity*, due to the high risk of sedation-related airway obstruction.
- *Anticipated difficult airway:* Deep sedation in such patients may precipitate a respiratory or airway crisis before definitive airway control is established, particularly in a non–operating room or otherwise suboptimal environment.
- *Severe cardiopulmonary disease*, where even brief hypoventilation or hypotension may be poorly tolerated.

13.7 Procedural Selection for MAC

13.7.1 Well-Suited Procedures

- Ophthalmologic surgery (e.g., cataract extraction).
- Superficial vascular access or port placement.
- Minor plastic or dermatologic procedures.
- Endoscopy and interventional radiology with limited procedural discomfort.
- Procedures where local or regional anesthesia provides the primary analgesia and MAC supplements comfort.

13.7.2 Poorly Suited Procedures

- Major open abdominal or thoracic surgery.
- Procedures expected to cause severe pain without feasible regional anesthesia techniques.
- Long or complex operations with a high likelihood of significant blood loss or instability.
- Emergency trauma cases where rapid airway control and immobility are essential.

13.8 The Imperative of Readiness to Convert

The most critical feature of MAC is the constant readiness to escalate to general anesthesia. Common triggers for conversion include:

- Airway obstruction or hypoventilation despite basic rescue maneuvers.
- Patient intolerance—excessive anxiety, movement, or pain.
- Procedural escalation, unexpected duration/complexity, or major procedure-related complication.
- Hemodynamic instability or complications requiring deeper anesthesia.

For this reason, every MAC setup must include the same airway equipment, oxygen delivery systems (including the anesthesia machine in the room with oxygen and air gas supply), positive-pressure ventilation capability, and rescue drugs available as in a general anesthetic.

13.9 Risks and Complications

Although generally safe, MAC carries risks:

- Airway obstruction and hypoventilation, especially with deep sedation.
- Hypoxemia and hypercapnia.
- Aspiration if airway reflexes are blunted.
- Hemodynamic instability (e.g., hypotension and bradycardia).
- Awareness or recall if sedation is inadequate (this should be discussed ahead of time with the patient or surrogate when appropriate).

The anesthesiologist mitigates these risks through careful drug titration, supplemental oxygen, capnography, and readiness for airway intervention.

13.10 Monitoring in MAC

ASA monitoring standards apply fully during MAC:

- Continuous pulse oximetry.
- ECG monitoring.
- Non-invasive blood pressure every 5 min.
- Capnography (especially during moderate-to-deep sedation).
- Temperature monitoring for long cases.

This distinguishes MAC from procedural sedation delivered by non-anesthesiologists, where monitoring may be less comprehensive.

13.11 Conclusion

MAC is a sophisticated anesthetic service that integrates individualized sedation, comprehensive physiologic monitoring, and constant readiness to transition to general anesthesia. It differs fundamentally from simple sedation by requiring the continuous presence of an anesthesia professional skilled in advanced airway management and resuscitation.Careful patient and procedure selection are essential. Individuals with severe anxiety, cognitive impairment, language barriers, anticipated difficult airways, or significant cardiopulmonary disease may be poor candidates. Similarly, procedures that necessitate complete immobility, produce intense pain, or impose substantial physiologic stress are generally better managed under general anesthesia.

The defining feature of MAC is not the depth or "lightness" of sedation but preparedness—the capacity to guide patients safely across varying levels of sedation while maintaining vigilance and the ability to convert seamlessly to general anesthesia whenever patient safety demands it.

Key Takeaways

1. *MAC is distinct from simple sedation*: It represents a comprehensive anesthetic service provided exclusively by anesthesia professionals, integrating ASA-standard monitoring, individualized sedation, and the capability for immediate conversion to general anesthesia.
2. Patient safety depends on vigilance and preparedness rather than the depth of sedation. The anesthesia professional must continuously assess airway patency, ventilation, and hemodynamic stability, maintaining readiness for advanced airway intervention at any time.
3. Drug selection is guided by patient and procedural factors. Common agents include propofol, midazolam, dexmedetomidine, opioids, and ketamine, titrated to achieve comfort, amnesia, and analgesia while preserving spontaneous respiration and hemodynamic control.
4. Careful patient and procedure selection are essential. Ideal candidates are cooperative, medically stable patients undergoing minimally painful procedures; poor candidates include those with anticipated difficult airways, severe anxiety, cardiopulmonary disease, or high procedural stimulation.
5. The defining feature of MAC is readiness. Successful practice requires the same equipment, monitoring, and crisis management capability as general anesthesia, emphasizing the anesthesiologist's dual responsibility for comfort and safety.

Suggested Reading

1. https://www.asahq.org/standards-and-practice-parameters/statement-on-continuum-of-depth-of-sedation-definition-of-general-anesthesia-and-levels-of-sedation-analgesia.
2. Practice Guidelines for Moderate Procedural Sedation and Analgesia 2018. A Report by the American Society of Anesthesiologists Task Force on Moderate Procedural Sedation and Analgesia, the American Association of Oral and Maxillofacial Surgeons, American College of Radiology, American Dental Association, American Society of Dentist Anesthesiologists, and Society of Interventional Radiology. Anesthesiology. 2018;128(3):437–79.
3. https://www.asahq.org/standards-and-practice-parameters/statement-on-distinguishing-monitored-anesthesia-care-from-moderate-sedation-analgesia.
4. American Society of Anesthesiologists Task Force on Sedation and Analgesia by Non-Anesthesiologists. Practice guidelines for sedation and analgesia by non-anesthesiologists. Anesthesiology. 2002;96(4):1004–17.
5. Apfelbaum JL, Silverstein JH, Chung FF, et al. Practice guidelines for postanesthetic care. Anesthesiology. 2013;118(2):291–307.
6. https://www.asahq.org/standards-and-practice-parameters/standards-for-basic-anesthetic-monitoring.

14 Regional Anesthesia: Peripheral Nerve Blocks

14.1 Introduction

Regional anesthesia has transitioned from a niche technique to a central pillar of perioperative care. Peripheral nerve blocks (PNBs) are now routine in orthopedic, general, vascular, and oncologic surgery. They may serve as the sole anesthetic in select cases, replace neuraxial techniques when contraindicated, or supplement general anesthesia to optimize pain control.

Most PNBs today are performed under ultrasound guidance, which enhances the accuracy of needle placement and reduces the risk of vascular puncture and local anesthetic systemic toxicity (LAST), the complications inherently associated with any technique involving local anesthetic administration. The reduced risk of LAST observed with routine use of ultrasound guidance likely reflects improved precision of needle placement, avoidance of inadvertent intravascular injection, and the use of lower total local anesthetic doses owing to more accurate perineural deposition. However, ultrasound does not reduce complication rates to zero; risks such as nerve injury, pneumothorax, LAST, and bleeding remain. Nerve blocks can be performed as single injections or with placement of a perineural catheter, through which either intermittent boluses or continuous infusions may be administered. Continuous nerve catheters provide the advantage of prolonged and often superior analgesia compared to single-injection techniques. However, their use introduces additional considerations, including the risk of bleeding, catheter migration (which may result in inadequate analgesia or, if vascular migration occurs, an increased risk of LAST), and infection. A commercially available peripheral nerve catheter kit is illustrated in Fig. 14.1. Furthermore, they require greater resources and expertise to manage effectively in the perioperative and postoperative setting. It should be noted that this chapter is not a comprehensive review of all nerve blocks but rather a focused discussion of the most used and clinically relevant techniques encountered in perioperative practice.

A. Mirrakhimov, *Anesthesiology Demystified for the Internist*,
https://doi.org/10.1007/978-3-032-16811-5_14

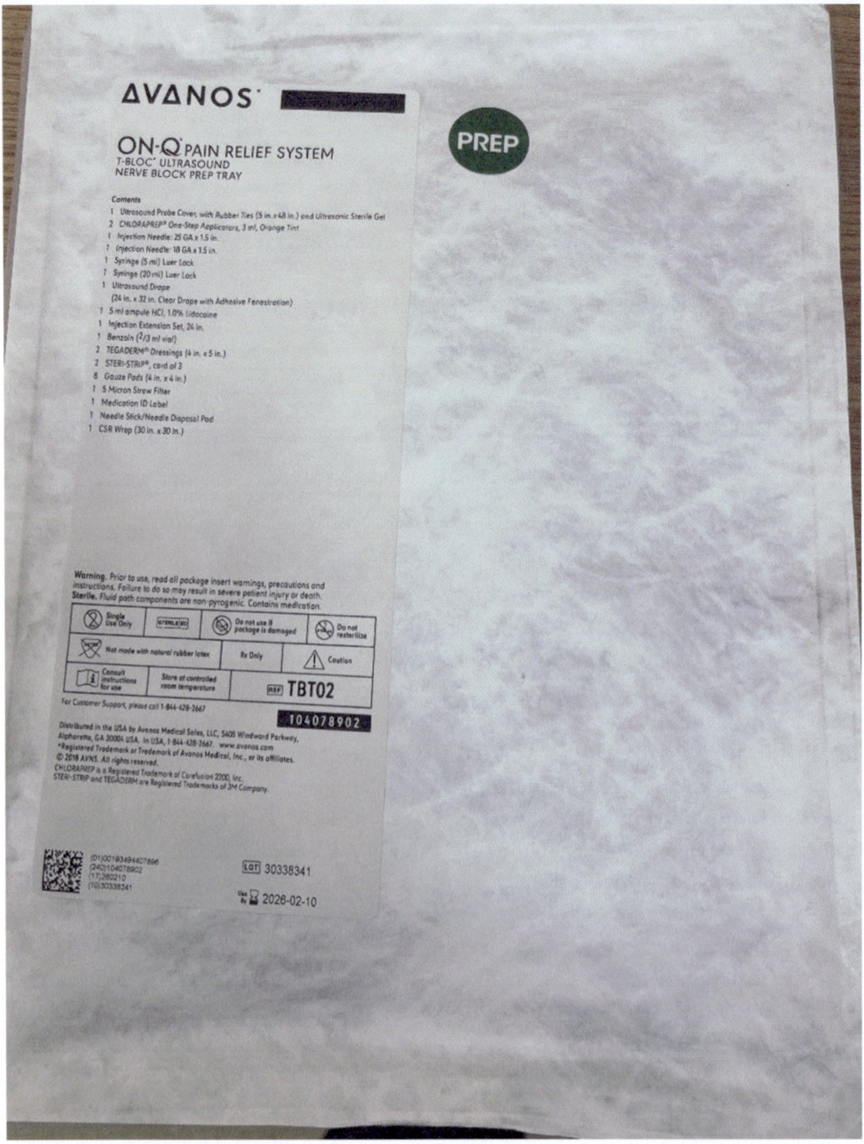

Fig. 14.1 Commercially available nerve catheter kit

For internists co-managing surgical patients, understanding PNBs provides context for postoperative findings (e.g., transient motor weakness, Horner's syndrome, and diaphragmatic dysfunction, among potential others), anticoagulation risk management, and multimodal analgesia pathways.

14.2 The Importance of Ultrasound in Regional Anesthesia

The introduction of ultrasound has revolutionized regional anesthesia and is now considered the standard of care for most PNBs. Traditional landmark-based and nerve stimulator-guided techniques relied on surface anatomy, paresthesia, or motor responses, which often led to variability in success rates and a higher risk of complications.

Ultrasound provides real-time visualization of nerves, surrounding structures (e.g., vessels, pleura, fascia, etc.), and the distribution of local anesthetic during injection. This capability improves accuracy, reduces the need for repeated needle passes, and enhances patient comfort. By lowering the likelihood of vascular puncture, lung injury (e.g., with some brachial plexus blocks, intercostal, paravertebral, and erector spinae plane (ESP) blocks), and intraneural injection, ultrasound reduces the incidence of LAST and improves overall safety. A still image of an ultrasound-guided pecto-intercostal fascial plane block for post-cardiac surgery analgesia is shown in Fig. 14.2.

Clinical studies demonstrate that ultrasound-guided blocks achieve faster onset, higher success rates, and longer duration of analgesia compared with older techniques. Additionally, ultrasound facilitates safer block placement in patients with obesity and distorted anatomy.

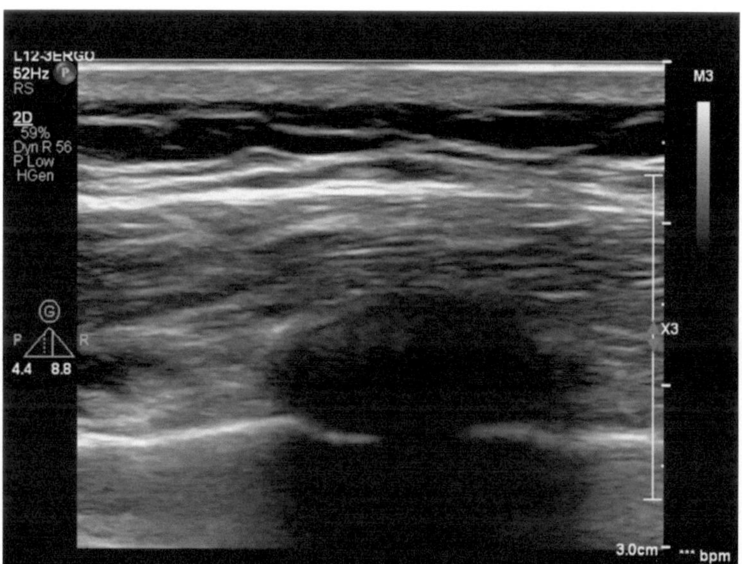

Fig. 14.2 A still image of an ultrasound-guided pecto-intercostal fascial plane block for post-cardiac surgery analgesia.

Despite these advantages, ultrasound is not infallible. Nerve injury, pneumothorax, bleeding, and infection can still occur, underscoring the need for formal training, anatomical knowledge, and vigilance. Nonetheless, ultrasound has transformed regional anesthesia into a more precise, effective, and safer practice, solidifying its role as a cornerstone of modern anesthesiology.

14.3 Truncal Versus Plexus/PNBs

- *Plexus and* PNB*s*: These include brachial plexus approaches (e.g., interscalene, supraclavicular, infraclavicular, axillary, etc.), lumbosacral plexus blocks (e.g., femoral, sciatic, lumbar plexus, etc.), and targeted distal nerve blocks (e.g., median nerve block, radial nerve block, etc.). They are most used for extremity surgery.
- *Truncal and fascial plane blocks*: These include transversus abdominis plane (TAP), rectus sheath, erector spinae plane (ESP), and paravertebral blocks. They provide wide dermatomal analgesia for thoracic or abdominal procedures, usually as analgesic adjuncts rather than primary surgical anesthesia.

14.4 Surgical Versus Analgesic/Adjunct Blocks

- *Surgical blocks*: Provide dense anesthesia sufficient for surgery without general anesthesia (e.g., brachial plexus blocks for hand surgery and femoral and sciatic nerve blocks for foot surgery). Surgical blocks are especially useful in patients where general anesthesia is undesirable. However, patient selection matters: factors such as severe anxiety, inability to tolerate an awake procedure, significant coagulopathy, or complex anatomy may limit suitability.
- *Analgesic/adjunct blocks*: Provide pain relief in conjunction with general anesthesia, often in enhanced recovery after surgery pathways (e.g., TAP block for laparoscopic surgery and ESP block for post-thoracotomy analgesia).

It is important to note that patients undergoing surgery with a nerve block as a primary anesthetic frequently receive intraprocedural sedation (e.g., midazolam, propofol, dexmedetomidine, etc.). This resembles monitored anesthesia care (MAC) but technically differs because the block provides the primary anesthetic, and the sedation only supplements patient comfort (e.g., anxiety, intraoperative noise, etc.).

14.5 Common PNBs

14.5.1 Brachial Plexus Blocks

14.5.1.1 Interscalene Block

- *Indications*: Shoulder, clavicle, and proximal humerus surgery.
- *Complications*: Almost universal ipsilateral phrenic nerve block; avoid in patients with significant pulmonary disease. Horner's syndrome and recurrent laryngeal

nerve block are possible. Lower risk of pneumothorax compared to supraclavicular and infraclavicular blocks. Vascular injury and bleeding.

14.5.1.2 Supraclavicular Block

- *Indications*: Upper extremity surgery distal to the shoulder.
- *Advantages*: Dense anesthesia and rapid onset.
- *Risks*: Pneumothorax (though reduced with ultrasound), occasional phrenic nerve involvement, vascular injury, and bleeding.

14.5.1.3 Infraclavicular Block

- *Indications*: Elbow, forearm, and hand surgery.
- *Advantages*: Reliable coverage of cords; catheter placement is feasible.
- *Risks*: Vascular injury and bleeding. Lower risk of phrenic nerve blockade compared to the supraclavicular block.

14.5.1.4 Axillary Brachial Plexus Block

- *Indications*: Surgery of the forearm and hand.
- *Advantages*: This approach represents a safer alternative to the aforementioned brachial plexus blocks, as it avoids phrenic nerve blockade and the risk of pneumothorax. However, it requires multiple needle passes to anesthetize individual nerves.
- *Risks*: Vascular injury and bleeding (more compressible site compared to supraclavicular and infraclavicular block sites).
- *Limitations*: May require supplemental blockade of musculocutaneous or axillary nerves.

14.5.2 Lower Extremity Blocks

14.5.2.1 Femoral Nerve Block

- *Indications*: Anterior thigh, knee procedures.
- *Risks*: Quadriceps weakness → fall risk. Vascular injury and bleeding.

14.5.2.2 Adductor Canal Block

- *Indications*: Postoperative analgesia after knee surgery.
- *Advantages*: Preserves quadriceps strength compared to the femoral block. Vascular injury and bleeding.

14.5.2.3 Popliteal Sciatic Block

- *Indications*: Foot/ankle surgery.
- *Limitations*: Saphenous nerve supplementation is often needed. Vascular injury and bleeding.

14.5.2.4 Lumbar Plexus Block

- *Indications*: Hip and major thigh surgery.
- *Risks*: Retroperitoneal hematoma; avoid with anticoagulation.

14.5.3 Truncal Blocks

14.5.3.1 TAP Block

- Analgesia for lower abdominal procedures. Simple, safe, opioid-sparing. There is an increased risk of LAST due to the large volume of local anesthetic required for this block.

14.5.3.2 Rectus Sheath Block

- For midline incisions; useful in hernia repair and pediatric surgery. There is an increased risk of LAST due to the large volume of local anesthetic required for this block.

14.5.3.3 ESP Block

- Provides broad thoracic or abdominal analgesia. Fewer complications; pneumothorax risk is rare but possible. There is an increased risk of LAST due to the large volume of local anesthetic required for this block.

14.5.3.4 Paravertebral Block

- Analgesia for breast, thoracic, and abdominal surgery. Unilateral somatic and sympathetic block. Risks include pneumothorax, hypotension, and vascular puncture.

14.6 Bleeding Risk and Anticoagulation

High-Risk (Deep, Non-compressible Blocks) Lumbar plexus, paravertebral, and infraclavicular

Lower-Risk (Superficial, Compressible Blocks) Femoral, axillary brachial plexus block, TAP, ESP, and rectus sheath.

American Society of Regional Anesthesia and Pain Medicine (ASRA) 2025 Guidelines

- Deep, non-compressible blocks should follow neuraxial-like anticoagulation precautions (e.g., paravertebral block).
- Superficial compressible blocks may be performed with less restriction, but clinical judgment and drug pharmacokinetics are critical for safe administration.
- Ultrasound guidance reduces but does not abolish bleeding risk.

14.7 Bier Block (Intravenous (IV) Regional Anesthesia)

- *Technique*: IV lidocaine after limb exsanguination and tourniquet inflation.
- *Indications*: Ideal for brief hand surgeries lasting less than 60 min.
- *Risks*: Tourniquet failure → systemic toxicity and seizures.
- *Modern role*: Largely limited due to alternatives.

14.8 Selection and Duration of Local Anesthetics (See Chap. 12 for More Information)

The choice of local anesthetic for PNB depends on the desired onset, duration, and safety profile relative to the surgical procedure and patient comorbidities. Short-acting agents such as chloroprocaine or lidocaine provide a rapid onset and are well-suited for brief procedures or when early neurologic assessment is desired. Intermediate-acting agents such as mepivacaine and prilocaine offer 2–3 hours of anesthesia, balancing onset and duration for moderate-length operations. Long-acting amide anesthetics—bupivacaine and ropivacaine—are most commonly used for surgical and postoperative analgesia, providing sensory blockade up to 6–18 hours after a single-shot technique, depending on concentration, site, and adjuncts.

Adjuncts such as *dexamethasone* and *dexmedetomidine* can further *prolong block duration* by modulating perineural inflammation and nerve conduction. Choice of local anesthetic also depends on toxicity profile; for example, ropivacaine is often preferred over bupivacaine because bupivacaine is associated with a higher risk of LAST and more refractory cardiovascular toxicity once LAST occurs. Continuous catheter techniques extend analgesia for several days but require careful monitoring.

Ultimately, local anesthetic selection should balance procedure length, desired sensory versus motor blockade, and patient safety.

14.9 Adjunct Agents for Regional Anesthesia

- *Dexamethasone*: Prolongs block duration (perineural or IV administration).
- *Dexmedetomidine*: Enhances block duration and quality; bradycardia/hypotension is possible.
- *Epinephrine*: Slows systemic uptake and modestly prolongs effect. Epinephrine is also used as a marker for inadvertent intravascular injection in certain regional anesthesia techniques, such as epidural anesthesia.
- *Sodium bicarbonate*: Alkalinizes local anesthetic solutions, hastening onset and reducing injection pain. Most effective with lidocaine; less used with long-acting amides due to precipitation risk.

14.10 Complications of PNBs

- LAST.
- Nerve injury (rare, often transient neuropraxia).
- Infection (rare with sterile technique).
- Block-specific risks: phrenic nerve block, pneumothorax, quadriceps weakness, and hematoma.
- Despite ultrasound guidance, complications do still occur.

14.11 Surgical Positioning and Airway Access

One often underappreciated factor in anesthesia planning is the patient's surgical position. Certain operations require post-induction positioning that restricts airway access, making anesthetic choice especially critical. For example, in shoulder surgery, patients are frequently placed in the beach chair position, which elevates the head and neck and rotates the torso. Once draped, airway access becomes challenging, and conversion from a failed block to general anesthesia may be very challenging. In such cases, anesthesiologists may favor secure airway management up front or ensure a surgical block with reliable coverage before positioning.

Similarly, hip arthroplasty is often performed in the lateral decubitus position, which can result in limited airway access due to surgical draping. If general anesthesia is chosen, securing the airway prior to turning is essential. Alternatively, combined spinal–epidural anesthesia or lumbar plexus/sciatic blocks may allow the procedure to proceed without airway instrumentation, provided the patient can tolerate remaining still.

Other examples include the prone position for spine surgery, which completely precludes airway access once surgery begins, and neurosurgical pin fixation for craniotomy, where even minor airway adjustments may be impossible after head fixation. In all these contexts, anesthesiologists weigh the reliability of regional anesthesia, patient comfort, comorbidities, and the anticipated need for airway intervention. For internists, awareness of these limitations clarifies why anesthesiologists may recommend against relying solely on certain blocks in patients at high risk for conversion to general anesthesia.

14.12 Conclusion

PNBs are versatile techniques that improve perioperative care by providing surgical anesthesia, postoperative analgesia, or both. The distinction between truncal and plexus blocks, surgical and purely analgesic blocks, as well as the associated anticoagulation-related bleeding risks, is critical for the safe and appropriate application of regional anesthesia techniques. Modern practice is largely ultrasound-guided, which improves accuracy and reduces but does not eliminate risks. Many blocks may serve as the primary anesthetic in select patients, though anxiety, comorbidities, or anatomy may limit candidacy. Patients often receive light intraprocedural sedation, similar in appearance to MAC, though technically distinct when the block provides the anesthetic.

Adjuncts such as dexamethasone, dexmedetomidine, epinephrine, and sodium bicarbonate extend block duration, quality, or comfort. For internists, understanding these techniques provides insight into perioperative management, anticoagulation considerations under ASRA guidance, and postoperative expectations.

Key Takeaways

1. PNBs may provide surgical anesthesia or analgesia, with truncal blocks mainly adjunctive and plexus blocks often suitable for complete surgical anesthesia.
2. Ultrasound guidance has become standard, improving accuracy, reducing complications, and enhancing block quality, though not eliminating risks.
3. ASRA 2025 guidelines recommend neuraxial-like caution for deep, non-compressible blocks in anticoagulated patients, while superficial blocks are generally safer.
4. Patients under nerve block anesthesia often receive light sedation, resembling MAC but distinct since the block provides the anesthetic.
5. Local anesthetic adjuncts (dexamethasone, dexmedetomidine, epinephrine, and sodium bicarbonate) enhance block onset, duration, and comfort, but require knowledge of risks.

Suggested Reading

1. Neal JM, Barrington MJ, Brull R, et al. The third ASRA practice advisory on neurologic complications associated with regional anesthesia. Reg Anesth Pain Med. 2015;40(5):401–30.
2. Kopp SL, Vandermeulen E, McBane RD et al. Regional anesthesia in the patient receiving antithrombotic or thrombolytic therapy: American Society of Regional Anesthesia and Pain Medicine Evidence-Based Guidelines (5th ed.). Reg Anesth Pain Med. 2025:rapm-2024-105766.
3. Taylor A, McLeod G. Basic pharmacology of local anesthetics. BJA Educ. 2020;20(2):34–41.
4. Becker DE, Reed KL. Local anesthetics: review of pharmacological considerations. Anesth Prog. 2012;59(2):90–101.
5. Mian A, Chaudhry I, Huang R, et al. Brachial plexus anesthesia: a review of the relevant anatomy, complications, and anatomical variations. Clin Anat. 2014;27(2):210–21.
6. Tran DQH, Elgueta MF, Aliste J, et al. Diaphragm-sparing nerve blocks for shoulder surgery. Reg Anesth Pain Med. 2017;42(1):32–8.
7. Tran DQ, Salinas FV, Benzon HT, et al. Lower extremity regional anesthesia: essentials of our current understanding. Reg Anesth Pain Med. 2019:rapm-2018-000019.
8. Chin KJ, Malhas L, Perlas A. The erector spinae plane block provides visceral abdominal analgesia in bariatric surgery: a report of 3 cases. Reg Anesth Pain Med. 2017;42(3):372–6.
9. Barrington MJ, Kluger R. Ultrasound guidance reduces risk of LAST after PNB. Reg Anesth Pain Med. 2013;38(4):289–99.

10. Eochagáin AN, Carolan S, Buggy DJ. Regional anaesthesia truncal blocks for acute postoperative pain and recovery: a narrative review. Br J Anaesth. 2024;132(5):1133–45.
11. Faccenda KA, Finucane BT. Complications of regional anesthesia. Drug Saf. 2001;24(6):413–42.

15 Neuraxial Anesthesia: Spinal, Epidural, and Combined Techniques

15.1 Introduction

Neuraxial anesthesia encompasses spinal, epidural, and combined spinal-epidural (CSE) techniques. These methods involve the injection of local anesthetics, often with adjuncts, into or around the cerebrospinal fluid (CSF) to interrupt nerve conduction at the spinal cord and nerve root levels.

- *Spinal anesthesia*: Direct injection of small volumes of local anesthetic into the subarachnoid space, producing rapid, dense, and predictable anesthesia. The commercially available spinal kit is shown in Fig. 15.1. Before reaching the spinal cord, a needle passes sequentially through the skin, subcutaneous tissue, supraspinous ligament, interspinous ligament, and ligamentum flavum, followed by the epidural space and then the dura mater and arachnoid mater. The spinal cord itself is protected within the subarachnoid space, which contains cerebrospinal fluid.
- *Epidural anesthesia*: Epidural anesthesia involves placement of a catheter into the epidural space using the tactile feedback of a loss-of-resistance syringe. This technique allows administration of larger volumes of local anesthetic and/or opioids, providing titratable and prolonged anesthesia or analgesia. A commercially available epidural kit is shown in Fig. 15.2, and a loss-of-resistance syringe is shown in Fig. 15.3. The epidural space is a potential space within the spinal canal located outside the dura mater, where local anesthetics and adjunct medications are injected. Medications administered into this space block spinal nerve roots, providing segmental analgesia or anesthesia while minimizing systemic drug exposure.
- *CSE*: A hybrid technique that provides the rapid onset of spinal anesthesia with the flexibility of epidural extension.

These approaches are widely used in orthopedic, vascular, lower abdominal, urologic, gynecologic, and obstetric surgery, as well as for acute and chronic pain management.

A. Mirrakhimov, *Anesthesiology Demystified for the Internist*,
https://doi.org/10.1007/978-3-032-16811-5_15

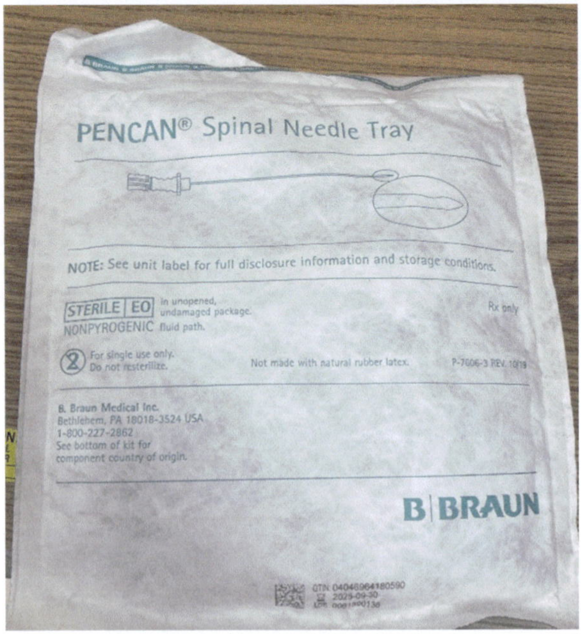

Fig. 15.1 Commercially available spinal kit

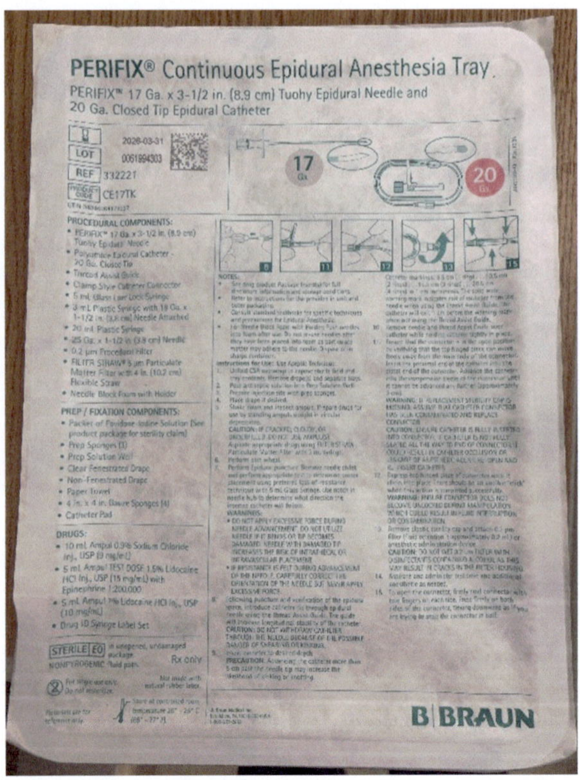

Fig. 15.2 Commercially available epidural kit

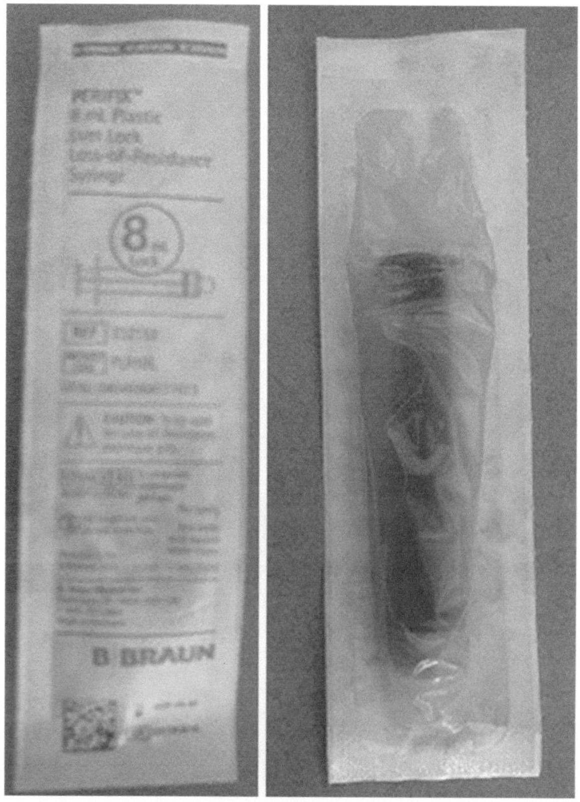

Fig. 15.3 Commercially available loss-of-resistance syringe

15.2 Dermatomes and Neuraxial Level Placement

Knowledge of dermatomal distribution is fundamental to neuraxial anesthesia. The spinal cord segments correspond to predictable cutaneous sensory levels: T4 approximates the nipples, T6 the xiphoid process, T10 the umbilicus, and L1 the inguinal ligament. For lower abdominal surgery, a block to at least T6–T8 is usually required, whereas cesarean delivery requires T4 coverage.

Epidural level placement is chosen to achieve a spread appropriate to the surgical site: lumbar epidurals for lower extremity/abdominal procedures and thoracic epidurals for thoracic or upper abdominal surgery.

15.3 Baricity of Local Anesthetics

Baricity describes the relative density of local anesthetics compared to CSF, influencing block distribution.

- *Hyperbaric solutions* (denser than CSF, often mixed with dextrose): Spread under gravity, allowing control via patient positioning.
- *Hypobaric solutions* (less dense than CSF): When injected intrathecally, a hypobaric solution rises against gravity, spreading toward non-dependent (higher) areas of the spinal canal.
- *Isobaric solutions* (same density as CSF): Spread more predictably, less position dependent. Isobaric solutions tend to remain near the injection site.

15.4 Indications

Surgical Blocks Lower abdominal, pelvic, urologic, lower extremity orthopedic, vascular, and cesarean delivery.

Analgesic Labor, postoperative pain (thoracotomy, laparotomy), and trauma (rib fractures).

15.5 Physiologic Effects and Risks of Sympathectomy

The hallmark physiologic effect of neuraxial anesthesia is sympathetic blockade, which becomes clinically significant when the block extends to the T4–T6 dermatomal levels, as this can produce notable decreases in systemic vascular resistance, venous return, and arterial blood pressure.

- *Cardiac*: Hypotension, bradycardia, and decreased preload and afterload.
- *Respiratory*: High blocks impair intercostal muscles; the diaphragm is preserved unless the block reaches the C3–C5 level.
- *Gastrointestinal (GI)/genitourinary (GU)*: Increased peristalsis and urinary retention.

15.6 Patients Not Ideal for Neuraxial Techniques Aiming at Surgical Block

Certain patient factors can make neuraxial anesthesia unsuitable or high risk when used as the primary surgical anesthetic technique. These include conditions that increase the likelihood of block failure, hemodynamic instability, bleeding, or neurologic complications, as well as circumstances where patient cooperation or positioning cannot be safely achieved. Some of the examples are provided below.

- *Severe aortic/mitral stenosis and hypertrophic cardiomyopathy*: Cannot tolerate reduced preload/systemic vascular resistance (SVR). Slow controlled epidural titration is often appropriate with strict hemodynamic monitoring (e.g., invasive blood pressure monitoring).
- *Pulmonary arterial hypertension (PAH) and RV dysfunction*: Risk of right ventricle (RV) failure with systemic vasodilation.
- *Severe hypovolemia*: Exacerbates shock.
- *Surgical positioning* (prone and lateral): Limits airway rescue.

15.7 Neurologic Disease Contraindications

- *Increased intracranial pressure (ICP) from mass lesion*: Herniation risk. Epidural anesthesia is not absolutely contraindicated in such patients; however, a significant risk remains if inadvertent dural puncture occurs.
- *Multiple sclerosis*: Controversial; potential relapse.
- *Pre-existing neuropathy*: Hard to assess new deficits.

15.8 Contraindications (General)

Absolute Patient refusal, local infection, systemic sepsis, severe hypovolemia, increased ICP, and local anesthetic (LA) allergy. If a patient has a suspected allergy to a local anesthetic, an alternative agent from a different class (e.g., an amide instead of an ester, or vice versa) may be considered after an appropriate evaluation.

Relative Anticoagulation, fixed cardiac output lesions (e.g., severe aortic stenosis), spinal deformity, and pre-existing neurologic disease.

15.9 Anticoagulation and Neuraxial Anesthesia

The following are general considerations, but the final decision regarding the safety and appropriateness of neuraxial anesthesia rests with the clinical judgment and expertise of the responsible anesthesiologist.

- *Aspirin/non steroidal antiinflammatory drugs (NSAIDs)*: Not contraindicated.
- *P2Y12 inhibitors*: Hold 5–7 days.
- *Warfarin*: International normalized ratio (INR) ≤1.4.
- *Unfractionated heparin (UFH)*: Wait 4–6 h.
- *Low molecular weight heparin (LMWH)*: ≥12 h prophylactic; ≥24 h therapeutic.
- *Direct oral anticoagulant (DOACs)*: Hold 2–5 days depending on renal function.
- *Neuraxial catheters*: Avoid during therapeutic anticoagulation.

15.10 Logistics of Neuraxial Techniques

15.10.1 Spinal Anesthesia

- *Onset*: 2–5 minutes and duration: 45–240 minutes (depending on the local anesthetic used).
- *Advantages*: Rapid, dense, reliable.
- *Disadvantages*: Limited duration (unless an intrathecal catheter is present), post-dural puncture headache (PDPH), high spinal, and hypotension.

15.10.2 Epidural Anesthesia

- *Onset*: 10–20 minutes (depending on the local anesthetic used). Duration: prolonged with a catheter.
- *Advantages*: Adjustable, titratable, long-term analgesia.
- *Disadvantages*: Technically harder to place, less dense block compared with spinal, and systemic toxicity risk (because higher doses of local anesthetics are usually needed).

15.10.3 CSE

- *Advantages*: Fast onset + prolonged flexibility.
- *Indications*: Labor, cesarean, orthopedic.
- *Risks*: Complications of both.

15.11 Neuraxial Adjuncts

Adjuncts enhance block or analgesia:

- *Morphine (hydrophilic, preservative-free)*: Prolonged analgesia (up to 12–24 hours), but risk of delayed respiratory depression, pruritus, and nausea.
- *Fentanyl (lipophilic)*: Rapid onset, shorter duration; improves block quality.
- *Clonidine (α2-agonist, preservative-free)*: Prolongs block, enhances analgesia, but may cause sedation and hypotension.
- *Epinephrine*: Added to local anesthetics to prolong duration (via vasoconstriction and reduced uptake of local anesthetic), reduce systemic absorption (lower local anesthetic systemic toxicity (LAST) risk), and serve as an intravascular marker if tachycardia occurs after test dose (to signify intravascular misplacement). Risks include ischemia (especially in patients with compromised spinal cord circulation).
- *Risks*: Use of non-preservative-free formulations has been linked to arachnoiditis and neurotoxicity.

15.12 Intrathecal Catheters

Intrathecal catheters may be placed intentionally (e.g., continuous spinal anesthesia in obstetrics or frail elderly patients needing titratable dosing) or unintentionally (misplacement during attempted epidural).

- *Benefits (intentional use)*: Ability to titrate doses, avoid repeat punctures, and manage high-risk patients with small incremental dosing.
- *Risks*: Catastrophic dosing errors if mistaken for an epidural catheter because intrathecal dosing volumes and drug dosages are 5–10 times lower. This can lead to total spinal anesthesia, hemodynamic collapse, and cardiorespiratory arrest. Intrathecal catheters are also associated with increased infectious risk.
- *Best practice*: Catheters must be clearly labeled, all staff informed, and strict protocols enforced.

15.13 High Spinal Anesthesia

A "high spinal" occurs when excessive local anesthetic spreads cephalad in the CSF.

Clinical Features
- Early: Numbness/weakness in arms and dyspnea.
- Progression: Hypotension, bradycardia (T1–T4 block), and respiratory compromise (C3–C5 involvement).
- Severe: Loss of consciousness and cardiovascular and respiratory collapse.

Management
- Immediate airway support (e.g., bag-mask ventilation, and intubation if necessary).
- IV fluids and vasopressors (e.g., norepinephrine, ephedrine, phenylephrine, etc.)
- Atropine or epinephrine for severe bradycardia/ and advanced cardiac life support.
- Supportive care until the block regresses.

15.14 PDPH

PDPH is a well-recognized complication of spinal anesthesia and inadvertent dural puncture during epidural placement. It is thought to result from persistent leakage of CSF through the dural hole, leading to decreased intracranial pressure and traction on pain-sensitive meningeal structures.

Clinical Features Typically occurs within 24–72 hours after puncture. The hallmark is a postural headache, worsening when upright and relieved by lying flat. It is often accompanied by neck stiffness, photophobia, nausea, and occasionally cranial nerve palsies (especially the VI cranial nerve).

Risk Factors

- Use of large or cutting-tip needles (e.g., Quincke and wet tap with epidural needle).
- Young age (higher risk in the obstetric population).
- Female gender.
- Low body mass index.
- Multiple puncture attempts.

Management:

- *Conservative measures*: Bed rest, hydration, caffeine, and analgesics may provide partial relief but do not reliably resolve symptoms.
- *Definitive treatment*: Epidural blood patch (injection of 15–20 mL autologous blood obtained in a sterile manner into the epidural space near the site of dural puncture) is the gold standard, sealing the dural leak and relieving symptoms in >90% of cases (some patients may need more than one epidural blood patch).
- *Other options*: Epidural saline, fibrin glue, sphenopalatine block, or pharmacologic therapies (e.g., theophylline and cosyntropin) in selected cases.

Preventive strategies include using smaller, pencil-point needles (e.g., Whitacre and Sprotte) for spinal anesthesia and minimizing the number of attempts.

15.15 Conclusion

Neuraxial anesthesia is foundational in modern anesthetic practice. Its benefits include profound surgical anesthesia and superior analgesia, but patient selection and vigilance are essential. Sympathectomy at T4–T6 underlies most hemodynamic changes. Adjuncts such as opioids, clonidine, and epinephrine expand utility but add risks. Intrathecal catheters provide flexibility yet demand strict safety protocols to avoid catastrophic dosing errors. Recognition and prompt treatment of complications such as high spinal anesthesia are critical for safe practice. For internists, awareness of contraindications and the physiological implications of neuraxial anesthesia enhances collaboration and patient-centered care.

Key Takeaways

1. Sympathectomy becomes clinically significant at T4–T6, producing hypotension and bradycardia.
2. Adjuncts (e.g., morphine, fentanyl, clonidine, and epinephrine) improve block quality but carry risks such as delayed respiratory depression and ischemia.
3. Intrathecal catheters must be clearly labeled to avoid dosing errors that can cause total spinal anesthesia.

4. High spinal requires immediate airway, hemodynamic, and pharmacologic support.
5. The American Society of Regional Anesthesia and Pain Medicine 2025 guidelines define strict anticoagulation management to prevent epidural hematoma.

Suggested Reading

1. Neal JM, Barrington MJ, Brull R, et al. The third ASRA practice advisory on neurologic complications associated with regional anesthesia. Reg Anesth Pain Med. 2015;40(5):401–30.
2. Kopp SL, Vandermeulen E, McBane RD et al. Regional anesthesia in the patient receiving antithrombotic or thrombolytic therapy: American Society of Regional Anesthesia and Pain Medicine Evidence-Based Guidelines (5th ed.). Reg Anesth Pain Med. 2025:rapm-2024-105766.
3. Uppal V, Russell R, Sondekoppam R, et al. Consensus practice guidelines on postdural puncture headache from a multisociety, international working group: a summary report. JAMA Netw Open. 2023;6(8):e2325387.
4. https://www.asahq.org/standards-and-practice-parameters/statement-on-neurologic-complications-of-neuraxial-analgesia-anesthesia-in-obstetrics.
5. https://www.nysora.com/techniques/spinal-anesthesia-2/.
6. https://www.nysora.com/topics/abdomen/epidural-anesthesia-analgesia/.
7. https://www.nysora.com/topics/abdomen/combined-spinal-epidural-anesthesia/.
8. Brenna CTA, Khan S, Poots C, et al. Association between perioperative neuraxial local anesthetic neurotoxicity and arachnoiditis: a narrative review of published reports. Reg Anesth Pain Med. 2024;49(10):726–50.
9. https://www.nysora.com/anesthesia/high-or-total-spinal-anesthesia/.

General Anesthesia: Induction, Maintenance, and Emergence

16

16.1 Introduction

General anesthesia (GA) is one of the most complex and finely tuned interventions in medicine. Unlike regional or neuraxial techniques, GA renders the patient completely unconscious, analgesic, and immobile. It is often the anesthetic of necessity when surgical invasiveness, patient comorbidities, or operative site preclude safe alternatives. A common preprocedural setup for GA is shown in Fig. 16.1.

The anesthetic state is not a single entity, but a dynamic continuum achieved and maintained by multiple pharmacologic agents. Anesthetic practice is structured into three main phases:

1. *Induction*: Transition from awake to anesthetized state.
2. *Maintenance*: Sustaining anesthesia during surgery, while managing physiological perturbations.

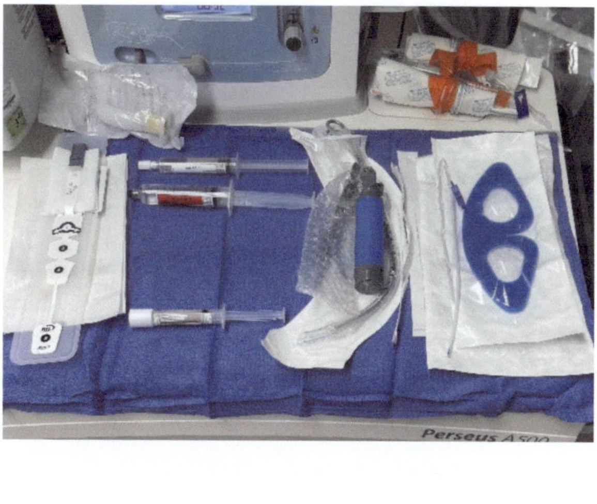

Fig. 16.1 Common preprocedural setup for GA. Note laryngoscopy blade, endotracheal tube (ETT), eye goggles for corneal protection, and intravenous catheter start kits

A. Mirrakhimov, *Anesthesiology Demystified for the Internist*,
https://doi.org/10.1007/978-3-032-16811-5_16

3. *Emergence*: Safe transition from anesthetized to awake state, with restoration of spontaneous breathing and airway reflexes. Certain patients, for example, those who are critically ill, recovering from cardiac surgery, or are anticipated to return to the operating room soon, may remain intubated at the end of the procedure.

16.2 Indications for GA

GA is indicated when:

- *Surgical requirements*: Procedures involving the thorax, abdomen, brain, spine, or other sites where absolute immobility is required.
- *Airway management*: Operations where the airway must be secured against aspiration (e.g., bowel obstruction and trauma).
- *Patient comfort and amnesia*: Long or painful procedures are often not feasible under regional anesthesia.
- *Contraindications to regional technique*: Coagulopathy, infection at the puncture site, or patient refusal.
- *Emergencies*: Trauma, hemorrhage, or compromised airway where rapid control is mandatory.

16.3 Choice of Airway Devices

16.3.1 Endotracheal Tube (ETT)

Pros
- Mechanical ventilation with the sealed airway (ETT cuff).
- Facilitates specialized procedures (lung isolation with double-lumen tubes, laser-resistant tubes which are used in some otorhinolaryngological surgeries, cuffed vs. uncuffed options). A commercially available double-lumen tube is shown in Fig. 16.2.

Cons
- Requires laryngoscopy, risk of airway trauma, hemodynamic stimulation, and dental injury.
- More invasive, higher incidence of sore throat, and hoarseness.

16.3.2 Laryngeal Mask Airway (LMA)

Pros
- Easier placement and less hemodynamic stress.
- Useful in short, low-risk procedures.
- Maintains spontaneous ventilation in select cases.

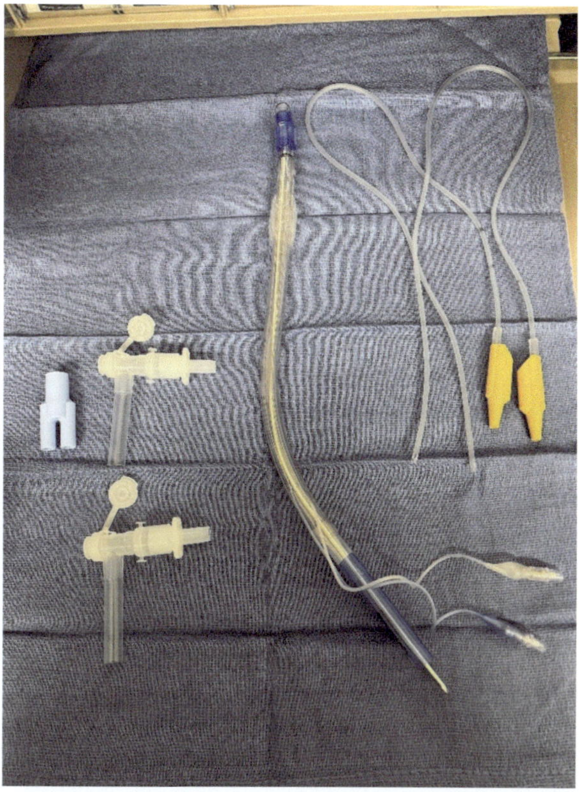

Fig. 16.2 Commercially available double-lumen ETT equipped with a tube connector and specialized suction catheters

Cons

- Not protective against aspiration.
- Less effective at high airway pressures, as the seal may be lost, compromising ventilation and increasing the risk of gastric insufflation.
- Contraindicated in patients with high aspiration risk (e.g., obesity with symptomatic gastroesophageal reflux disease, bowel obstruction, etc.).

Clinical Principle The choice between LMA and ETT reflects a balance between surgical requirements, aspiration risk, patient physiology, and expected airway pressures. A commercially available double-lumen tube is shown in Fig. 16.3.

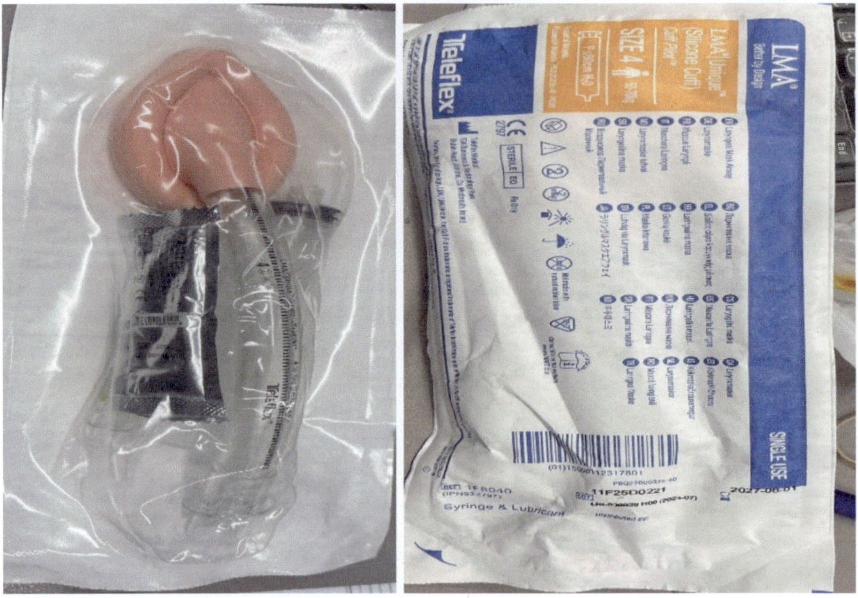

Fig. 16.3 A commercially available LMA

16.4 Induction of GA

Goals Achieve unconsciousness, amnesia, analgesia, and immobility while securing the airway and maintaining hemodynamic stability.

16.4.1 Pre-induction Preparation

- Pre-oxygenation to provide oxygen reserve.
- IV access, monitoring (American Society of Anesthesiologists (ASA) standards), and positioning.
- Rapid sequence induction should be considered when the risk of aspiration is high.

16.4.2 Agents Used

- *IV induction agents (see Chap. 11)*: Propofol (most commonly used, rapid onset, hypotension risk), etomidate (cardiac stability, adrenal suppression), ketamine (sympathomimetic, useful in trauma, PAH, asthmatics), and thiopental (rare in the United States, used abroad).
- *Adjuncts (see Chap. 12)*: Opioids (fentanyl, sufentanil, and remifentanil), IV lidocaine to blunt sympathetic response to laryngoscopy.

- *Neuromuscular blockers*: Succinylcholine (rapid onset, short duration, but risk of hyperkalemia, malignant hyperthermia) and rocuronium (longer duration, reversible with sugammadex).

16.4.3 Airway Management During Induction

- Direct laryngoscopy, video laryngoscopy, or supraglottic airway placement.
- Anesthesiologists must always be prepared for an unanticipated difficult airway.

16.5 Maintenance of GA

Techniques

- *Inhalational agents*: Sevoflurane, desflurane, isoflurane, and nitrous oxide. Allow titratable depth and rapid emergence with low-solubility agents.
- *Total intravenous anesthesia (TIVA)*: Propofol infusion, often with remifentanil; useful for neurosurgical procedures requiring neuromonitoring where inhaled agents suppress evoked potentials. TIVA without volatile agents is mandatory in patients with a personal or family history of malignant hyperthermia. Additionally, TIVA with propofol should be considered in patients with a history of postoperative nausea and vomiting who have failed to respond to conventional prophylactic measures in the past (see Chap. 25).
- *Balanced anesthesia*: A combination of inhaled agent, opioid, and neuromuscular blockade.

Goals

- Maintain unconsciousness, analgesia, and immobility.
- Optimize oxygen delivery and organ perfusion.
- Control hemodynamic responses to surgical stress.

16.6 Emergence From GA

Goals

- Restore spontaneous breathing and airway reflexes.
- Reverse neuromuscular blockade (neostigmine + glycopyrrolate, or sugammadex for aminosteroids).
- Ensure hemodynamic stability and normothermia.

Complications During Emergence

- Laryngospasm (risk is higher in the pediatric population) and airway obstruction.
- Hemodynamic lability (tachycardia, hypertension).
- Delirium or emergence agitation.
- Residual neuromuscular weakness and incomplete reversal → hypoxemia, hypercapnia, aspiration, and risk of reintubation.

16.7 Advanced Monitoring in GA

16.7.1 Arterial Line

- *Indications:* Major surgery with anticipated hemodynamic swings (cardiac, vascular, neurosurgery, and trauma), critically ill patients in shock, and patients with high-risk comorbid conditions (e.g., severe aortic stenosis and pulmonary arterial hypertension (PAH)).
- Provides beat-to-beat blood pressure and frequent labs (arterial blood gas (ABG) and lactate).
- *Complications:* hematoma, limb ischemia, and inadvertent medication administration.

16.7.2 Central Venous Catheter (CVC)

- *Indications:* Administration of vasoactive drugs, volume assessment, and difficult peripheral venous access.
- *Limitations:* Central venous pressure correlates poorly with intravascular volume status and should instead be interpreted as a dynamic trend rather than an absolute measure.
- *Complications*: Bleeding, accidental arterial injury and misplacement, air embolism, and pneumothorax.

16.7.3 Pulmonary Artery Catheter (PAC)

- *Indications:* Severe heart failure, complex cardiac surgery, PAH, and transplant surgery.
- Provides cardiac output, pulmonary artery pressures, and mixed venous oxygen saturation.
- *Complications*: In addition to the complications associated with CVC placement, additional risks include complete heart block, PAC entrapment, and pulmonary artery rupture—the latter representing a rare but catastrophic event.

16.7.4 Transesophageal Echocardiography (TEE)

- *Indications:* Cardiac surgery, thoracic aortic surgery, and hemodynamic instability of unclear cause.
- Provides real-time cardiac imaging, volume status, contractility, and valvular pathology. The TEE machine is shown in Fig. 16.4.
- *Complications:* Oropharyngeal trauma, loss of airway from inadvertent ETT dislodgement during placement, gastrointestinal bleeding, perforation, and probe entrapment.

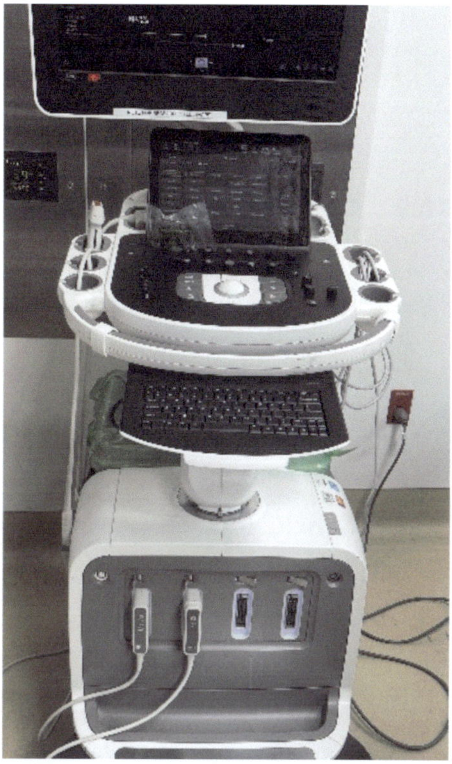

Fig. 16.4 Commercially available TEE machine

16.7.5 Neuromonitoring

- *NIRS (near-infrared spectroscopy)*: Monitors cerebral or somatic tissue oxygenation; used in cardiac and vascular surgery (e.g., carotid surgery or stenting).
- *SSEP/MEP (somatosensory and motor evoked potentials)*: Monitor spinal cord function during scoliosis or aortic surgery. Anesthetic implications: Inhaled agents and muscle relaxants depress signals; TIVA is preferred.
- *Electroencephalogram (EEG) and processed EEG (e.g., bispectral index (BIS))*: Used to titrate anesthetic depth and potentially reduce intraoperative awareness.
- *Clinical pearl*: Neuromonitoring frequently necessitates TIVA, which relies on dependable intravenous access. However, this technique carries a risk of intraoperative awareness if IV access becomes compromised or nonfunctional without prompt recognition. Unlike volatile anesthetics, IV agents lack an expired gas concentration for monitoring, limiting the ability to verify anesthetic delivery.

16.8 Anesthetic Implications of Neuromonitoring

- *SSEP*: Suppressed by volatile agents >0.5 minimum alveolar concentration; opioids and propofol are less disruptive.

- *MEP*: Extremely sensitive to anesthetics; TIVA with propofol/remifentanil is preferred. Neuromuscular blockade should be minimized.
- *EEG/BIS*: Guides anesthetic depth, especially during TIVA cases.
- *NIRS*: Guides hemodynamic management in cardiac/vascular procedures.

16.9 Complications of GA

- *Airway-related*: Trauma, laryngospasm, and aspiration.
- *Hemodynamic*: Hypotension, hypertension, and arrhythmias.
- *Respiratory*: Hypoxemia, hypercarbia, and bronchospasm.
- *Neurologic*: Awareness (rare), postoperative delirium, and cognitive dysfunction.
- *Others*: Malignant hyperthermia and anaphylaxis.

16.10 Conclusion

GA underpins the practice of modern anesthesiology and surgery. Induction, maintenance, and emergence must be individualized to patient comorbidities, surgical requirements, and monitoring needs. While ASA monitors form the foundation of safety, certain cases demand advanced monitoring such as arterial lines, CVC, PAC, TEE, and neuromonitoring. Each has distinct anesthetic implications.

Airway management is central: the LMA offers simplicity but limited protection against aspiration, while the ETT remains the gold standard for aspiration protection and high-pressure ventilation. Anesthesiologists must balance pharmacologic regimens, hemodynamic control, and neuromonitoring fidelity.

For internists, understanding these principles clarifies perioperative risk assessment, postoperative complications, and why anesthesiologists may advocate advanced monitoring or specific airway strategies. GA is not simply "putting the patient to sleep" but a highly dynamic, evidence-driven process integrating physiology, pharmacology, and technology to optimize patient safety.

Key Takeaways

1. GA provides unconsciousness, amnesia, analgesia, and immobility, delivered in phases: induction, maintenance, and emergence.
2. Airway choice (LMA vs. ETT) depends on aspiration risk, airway pressures, and surgical context.
3. Advanced monitoring (arterial line, CVC, PAC, TEE, and neuromonitoring) is reserved for high-risk patients or complex surgeries.
4. Neuromonitoring imposes anesthetic implications—volatile agents suppress SSEPs/MEPs, favoring TIVA in spine/cardiac cases.
5. Emergence is a vulnerable phase, with risks of laryngospasm, hemodynamic swings, and residual weakness.

Suggested Reading

1. Brown EN, Lydic R, Schiff ND. General anesthesia, sleep, and coma. N Engl J Med. 2010;363(27):2638–50.
2. Laferrière-Langlois P, Morisson L, Jeffries S. Depth of anesthesia and nociception monitoring: current state and vision for 2050. Anesth Analg. 2024;138(2):295–307.
3. Murkin JM, Arango M. Near-infrared spectroscopy as an index of brain and tissue oxygenation. Br J Anaesth. 2009;103(Suppl 1):i3–i13.
4. Deiner S. Highlights of anesthetic considerations for intraoperative neuromonitoring. Semin Cardiothorac Vasc Anesth. 2010;14(1):51–3.
5. Ryalino C, Sahinovic MM, Drost G, et al. Intraoperative monitoring of the central and peripheral nervous systems: a narrative review. Br J Anaesth. 2024;132(2):285–99.
6. Bartels K, Esper SA, Thiele RH. Blood pressure monitoring for the anesthesiologist: a practical review. Anesth Analg. 2016;122(6):1866–79.
7. de Keijzer IN, Scheeren TWL. Perioperative hemodynamic monitoring: an overview of current methods. Anesthesiol Clin. 2021;39(3):441–56.
8. Efrimescu CI, Moorthy A, Griffin M. Rescue transesophageal echocardiography: a narrative review of current knowledge and practice. J Cardiothorac Vasc Anesth. 2023;37(4):584–600.

Surgical Positioning: Techniques, Physiologic Implications, and Perioperative Risks

17

17.1 Introduction

Surgical positioning enables operative exposure, but it is never neutral for physiology. Venous return, cardiac output, pulmonary mechanics, cerebral perfusion, and tissue interface pressures all shift with position. Position also determines how easily the anesthesia team can see and reach the patient's face, airway, and monitors, which are the factors that directly influence rescue options when instability or airway failure occurs.

From an anesthetic perspective, optimal positioning is a shared responsibility: the surgeon defines exposure requirements; anesthesia anticipates physiological consequences and airway implications; and nursing and technologist teams ensure protective padding, neutral alignment, and pressure-point safety. High-reliability practice emphasizes checklists, pre-positioning briefings, continuous pressure and nerve-injury vigilance, and clear contingency plans (e.g., how to emergently flip a prone patient, when to abandon a position, etc.).

17.2 Core Principles of Safe Positioning

- *Protect perfusion and pressure*: Avoid prolonged pressure on bony prominences and soft tissues; distribute load; reposition when feasible.
- *Preserve neutral alignment*: Head/neck, shoulders, and hip/knee/ankle in neutral to reduce plexus and peripheral nerve stretch/compression.
- *Arms*: Prefer <90° abduction; forearm neutral or supinated to reduce the risk of ulnar nerve injury; careful padding at elbow and humerus.
- *Eyes*: No direct pressure; confirm eyelids taped and corneas protected in all positions, especially prone.
- *Cables/lines*: Free of tension; avoid loops under pressure points.

A. Mirrakhimov, *Anesthesiology Demystified for the Internist*,
https://doi.org/10.1007/978-3-032-16811-5_17

- *Hemodynamics and ventilation*: Anticipate position-related changes in venous return, lung compliance, and airway pressures; adjust ventilator and vasoactive strategy.
- *Airway access*: If intraoperative airway rescue would be delayed (prone, sitting with drapes, lateral with supports), strongly consider general anesthesia with a secured airway endotracheal tube (ETT) rather than deep sedation or regional technique alone.
- *Team briefing*: Pre-positioning timeout specifying pressure points, nerve risks, planned duration, rescue plan, and eye checks.

17.3 Supine Position

17.3.1 Technique and Indications

Most common position; suitable for abdominal, pelvic, vascular, and many orthopedic procedures. Arms may be tucked or abducted (<90°).

17.3.2 Physiological Implications

- *Hemodynamics*: Neutral to slight increase in venous return versus sitting or upright; obesity/pregnancy may still reduce functional residual capacity (FRC) and increase atelectasis risk.
- *Respiratory*: Decreased FRC compared with upright; dependent lung atelectasis is common under general anesthesia.

17.3.3 Risks and Complications

- *Peripheral nerve*: Ulnar neuropathy (elbow compression), brachial plexus stretch with excessive abduction, and radial/median compression at the distal humerus/forearm.
- *Pressure injuries*: Occiput, scapula, sacrum, and heels; pressure alopecia with long cases.

17.3.4 Prevention

Elbow padding, limit arm abduction, and neutral wrist/forearm; gel pads for occiput/heels; vigilance for prolonged cases.

17.4 Lateral Decubitus Position

17.4.1 Technique and Indications

Used for thoracic, renal, and hip surgeries. Upper arm supported; axillary roll placed under the thorax (not the axilla) to offload the dependent neurovascular bundle. Dependent knee flexed, nondependent leg extended with padding between knees/ankles.

17.4.2 Physiology

- *Hemodynamics*: Variable preload; venous return may decline with excessive table flexion.
- *Respiratory*: Marked ventilation/perfusion (V/Q) mismatch—dependent lung is better perfused but may be compressed; one-lung ventilation augments the mismatch.

17.4.3 Risks

- *Brachial plexus*: Stretch/compression from head/shoulder malalignment or arm abduction >90°.
- *Peroneal nerve*: Compression at the fibular head of the dependent leg.
- *Eye and ear*: Pressure injury to the dependent eye/auricle; corneal abrasion if the face is malpositioned.
- *Compartment pressure*: Dependent muscle groups at risk during long cases.

17.4.4 Prevention

Meticulous head/neck alignment; confirm proper axillary roll position (under the dependent chest, clearly below the axilla); check pulses/paresthesias (if not under general anesthesia) after final positioning; protect eyes and contralateral breast/pectoralis with gel; frequent re-checks.

17.5 Prone Position

17.5.1 Technique and Indications

Common for spine, posterior fossa cranial surgery, and select orthopedic procedures. Intubation is performed supine; the patient is then carefully turned prone with the head supported in a foam/gel headrest or pins (for neurosurgery). Abdomen is free to minimize the compression of the inferior vena cava; chest is supported.

17.5.2 Physiology

- *Hemodynamics*: Venous return can fall if the abdomen is compressed; increased intra-abdominal and intrathoracic pressures raise venous pressure and increase bleeding risk.
- *Respiratory*: Variable effects, chest wall compliance often decreases; positive end expiratory pressure (PEEP) may be needed to maintain oxygenation.

17.5.3 Risks

- *Airway*: Loss of airway access once prone; ETT dislodgement during turn; secretions pooling.
- *Perioperative visual loss*: Rare but catastrophic ischemic optic neuropathy or central retinal artery occlusion; risk rises with prolonged surgery, anemia, hypotension, large blood loss, high venous pressure, and direct eye pressure.
- *Peripheral nerve and pressure injury*: Brachial plexus (arm abduction >90°, shoulder roll malposition), ulnar nerve, and lateral femoral cutaneous nerve; breast/genital compression; pressure sores on face, chest, iliac crests, and knees.
- *Venous congestion/bleeding*: From abdominal compression.

17.5.4 Prevention

Secure ETT with bite block and robust fixation; coordinate a controlled team "turn"; confirm equal breath sounds and capnography after positioning; keep abdomen free; limit crystalloid; maintain hemoglobin and perfusion pressure; no direct eye pressure with periodic eye checks; document head/neck neutral, arms <90° abduction, and padding.

17.6 Steep Trendelenburg (Head-Down)

17.6.1 Technique and Indications

Common in laparoscopic/robotic pelvic surgery (gynecologic/urologic). Head down with shoulder braces or well-padded attachments.

17.6.2 Physiology

- *Hemodynamics*: Venous return increases; cardiac output may rise but can be limited by increased intrathoracic pressure from pneumoperitoneum.
- *Respiratory*: Marked drop in pulmonary compliance; increased airway pressures; atelectasis; higher risk of hypercarbia with pneumoperitoneum.
- *Neuro-ocular*: Increased intracranial and intraocular pressures intraocular pressure (IOP).

17.6.3 Risks

- *Airway/upper-body edema*: Facial, tongue, and laryngeal edema after long cases—postoperative stridor risk.
- *Brachial plexus*: Shoulder braces can compress/clavicle–first rib region; sliding can cause stretch.
- *Ocular*: Elevated IOP; theoretical ischemic optic risk in prolonged head-down states.
- *Rhabdomyolysis/compartment*: Rare in prolonged, high-pressure cases.

17.6.4 Prevention

Secure patient with nonslip mats and pelvis/torso straps instead of shoulder braces when possible; limit time/head-down angle; minimize fluids; periodic pneumoperitoneum/Trendelenburg breaks; consider leak-test or direct laryngoscopy in post operative care unit (PACU) for high-risk airway edema; eye protection.

17.7 Beach Chair/Sitting Position

17.7.1 Technique and Indications

Used for shoulder arthroscopy/open procedures and some posterior cranial cases. Head held neutral with a horseshoe support or pin fixation for neurosurgery; torso upright 30–70°.

17.7.2 Physiology

- *Hemodynamics*: Reduced venous return → hypotension risk; cerebral perfusion depends on arterial pressure at the circle of Willis, which is ~20–30 mmHg lower than cuff pressure at the arm when upright.
- *Respiratory*: Increased FRC versus supine; generally favorable mechanics.

17.7.3 Risks

- *Cerebral hypoperfusion*: Relative cerebral hypotension given the positioning. Cerebral perfusion pressure decreases by approximately 7.4 mmHg for every 10 cm the brain is positioned above the mid-axillary line at the level of the fourth intercostal space.
- *Venous air embolism (VAE)*: With non-collapsible venous sinuses in cranial surgery; less common in the shoulder, but possible during open procedures.

- *Brachial plexus/neck*: Stretch from shoulder traction or malposition; pressure on the nondependent peroneal nerve at the fibular head.
- *Pressure*: Gluteal/ischial and occipital pressure injuries.

17.7.4 Prevention

Measure blood pressure at the level of the brain (adjusted transducer height or cerebral oximetry guidance); avoid excessive deliberate hypotension; secure head/neck neutral; careful shoulder traction limits; consider precordial Doppler/ETCO_2 monitoring when VAE risk is significant; PEEP cautiously to reduce venous entrainment.

17.8 Head Pinning (Craniotomy and Cervical Spine)

17.8.1 Technique and Purpose

Three-point skull fixation (e.g., Mayfield pins) provides rigid head control for cranial and cervical procedures.

17.8.2 Implications and Risks

- *Hemodynamic reflexes*: Pin placement can cause abrupt hypertension and tachycardia; treat with adequate depth or local infiltration of local anesthetics.
- *Bleeding*: Scalp bleeds briskly; inspect pin sites; avoid coagulopathy.
- *VAE*: Sitting/craniotomy increases venous air entrainment risk through noncollapsible veins/sinuses.
- *Pressure/skin injury*: From pin torque on osteoporotic skull or improper placement.

17.8.3 Prevention and Monitoring

Deepen anesthesia or infiltrate local before pinning; confirm pin torque; monitor for VAE (ETCO_2 drop, precordial Doppler, transesophageal echocardiography (TEE) in select cases); communicate clearly before any head movement; protect eyes and avoid facial pressure.

17.9 Why General Anesthesia Is Often Selected When Airway Access Will Be Limited

When the patient's face and airway become inaccessible (e.g., prone, lateral with rigid supports, beach chair with sterile field and traction, and head pinning), the tolerance for airway uncertainty is low. Even brief hypoventilation, aspiration, or tube dislodgement can be catastrophic if rescue requires time-consuming repositioning or drape takedown. For this reason, anesthesiologists frequently prefer general anesthesia with a secured endotracheal tube and capnography rather than deep sedation or regional anesthesia alone. If regional anesthesia is used as a primary technique (e.g., interscalene block for shoulder surgery), it is often supplemented by secured airway or very light sedation with a fully rehearsed plan for conversion, recognizing that patient anxiety, surgical stimulation, or block failure may necessitate immediate airway control.

17.10 Conclusion

Surgical positioning is a major modifier of perioperative risk and physiology. Supine positioning is deceptively "simple," yet ulnar neuropathy and pressure injuries remain concerns. Lateral positioning challenges V/Q matching and exposes the brachial plexus and peroneal nerve to injury when alignment and padding are suboptimal. Prone positioning can compromise venous return, obscure the airway, and, in rare situations, be the cause of postoperative visual loss if perfusion and eye protection are not meticulously managed. Steep Trendelenburg improves pelvic exposure but increases airway and facial edema and ocular pressure. The beach chair/sitting position offers respiratory advantages but demands vigilance for cerebral hypoperfusion and VAE, with blood pressure interpreted at the brain's level. Head pinning for cranial and cervical procedures adds hemodynamic surges, bleeding, and air embolism considerations.

These risks underscore why anesthesiologists often prefer general anesthesia with a secured airway in cases where intraoperative access is expected to be limited or delayed. Ultimately, safe patient positioning is a team effort, which requires anticipation of physiological changes, protection of peripheral nerves, relief of soft tissue pressure, verification of ocular safety, and maintenance of a clear rescue plan. Consistent use of checklists, periodic reassessment, and open interdisciplinary communication are essential to minimizing preventable harm and promoting optimal outcomes.

Key Takeaways

1. *Position determines physiology*: Anticipate shifts in venous return, lung mechanics, and cerebral perfusion—and adjust ventilation and hemodynamics accordingly.
2. *Protect nerves and eyes*: Limit arm abduction, pad vulnerable points, maintain neutral alignment, and prevent direct ocular pressure—especially in the prone position.
3. *Head-down and beach chair carry distinct risks*: Expect airway/upper-body edema and ocular pressure with steep Trendelenburg. Protect cerebral perfusion (e.g., avoidance of hypotension) and monitor for VAE in beach chair/sitting.

4. *Airway strategy follows access*: When airway rescue will be difficult (prone, lateral with rigid supports, and head pinning), anesthesiologists favor general anesthesia with a secured endotracheal tube (ETT).
5. *Checklists and re-checks are essential:* Pre-position briefing, pressure-point/eye checks, proper leveling of monitors, and documented reassessment reduce complications.

Suggested Reading

1. Practice Advisory for the Prevention of Perioperative Peripheral Neuropathies 2018. An updated report by the American Society of Anesthesiologists Task Force on Prevention of Perioperative Peripheral Neuropathies. Anesthesiology. 2018;128(1):11–26.
2. Practice Advisory for Perioperative Visual Loss Associated with Spine Surgery 2019. An updated report by the American Society of Anesthesiologists Task Force on Perioperative Visual Loss, the North American Neuro-Ophthalmology Society, and the Society for Neuroscience in Anesthesiology and Critical Care. Anesthesiology. 2019;130(1):12–30.
3. Edgcombe H, Carter K, Yarrow S. Anaesthesia in the prone position. Br J Anaesth. 2008;100(2):165–83.
4. Pohl A, Cullen DJ. Cerebral ischemia during shoulder surgery in the upright position: a case series. J Clin Anesth. 2005;17(6):463–9.
5. Tufegdzic B, Lamperti M, Siyam A, et al. Air-embolism in the semi-sitting position for craniotomy: a narrative review with emphasis on a single centers experience. Clin Neurol Neurosurg. 2021;209:106904.
6. https://www.uptodate.com/contents/patient-positioning-for-surgery-and-anesthesia-in-adults.

Part V

Recovery, Complications, and Pain Management

18 Post-Anesthesia Care Unit: Structure, Assessment, and Discharge Criteria

18.1 Introduction

The recovery period following anesthesia and surgery is one of the most vulnerable phases of patient care. Patients emerging from anesthesia may experience residual sedation, impaired airway reflexes, unstable hemodynamics, inadequate pain control, nausea, or complications such as hypoxemia or arrhythmia. The post-anesthesia care unit (PACU) was established to provide structured monitoring during this high-risk transition.

The modern PACU typically functions as a specialized unit adjacent to the operating suite, staffed by trained nurses and supervised by anesthesiologists or other qualified physicians (see Fig. 18.1). Its mission is to provide early recognition and

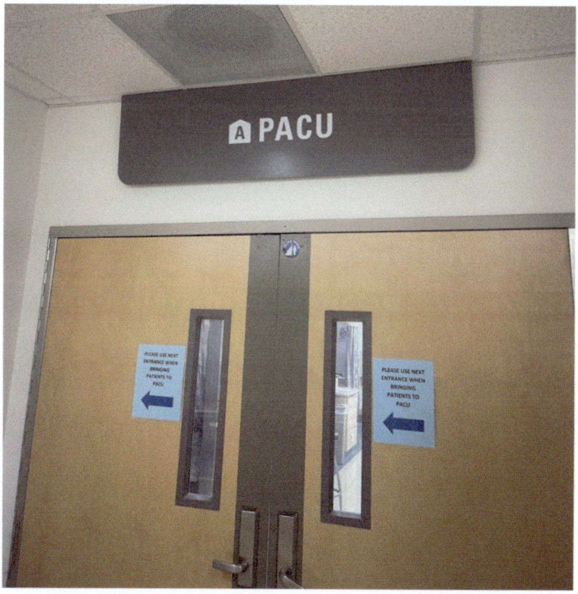

Fig. 18.1 PACU entrance at the University of Kentucky Albert Chandler Hospital

A. Mirrakhimov, *Anesthesiology Demystified for the Internist*,
https://doi.org/10.1007/978-3-032-16811-5_18

intervention for complications, smooth handoff from the operating room (OR) team, and determine readiness for safe discharge to the ward, home, or intensive care unit (ICU).

18.2 Structure of the PACU

18.2.1 Physical Layout

- *Proximity*: PACU should be located near operating rooms to allow rapid transport and return if re-intervention is necessary.
- *Bed spacing*: Each patient bay requires space for monitors, ventilators, infusion pumps, and immediate access by staff.
- *Monitors*: Standardized equipment includes ECG, non-invasive blood pressure, pulse oximetry, and often capnography for high-risk patients.
- *Emergency readiness*: Airway carts, defibrillators, and resuscitation equipment must be readily available.

18.2.2 Staffing

- *Nurses*: The backbone of PACU care; typically a 1:1 or 1:2 nurse-to-patient ratio during Phase I recovery.
- *Anesthesiologists*: Provide supervision, respond to complications, and approve discharges.
- *Surgeons*: Available for wound or surgical concerns.
- *Ancillary staff*: Respiratory therapists, pharmacists, and support personnel.

18.3 PACU Assessment

PACU assessment follows a structured approach emphasizing rapid detection of instability:

1. *Airway*: Patency, protective reflexes, evidence of obstruction, and secretions.
2. *Breathing*: Respiratory rate, tidal volume, oxygen saturation, and capnography when indicated.
3. *Circulation*: Heart rate, rhythm, blood pressure, and perfusion.
4. *Neurologic*: Level of consciousness, orientation, motor/sensory status (especially after regional anesthesia).
5. *Pain*: Subjective reports (numeric rating scale) and behavioral cues.
6. *Other*: Temperature, urine output, nausea/vomiting, and surgical site checks.

18.3.1 Common Problems Detected in PACU

- *Airway obstruction*: Tongue collapse and laryngospasm.
- *Respiratory compromise*: Hypoxemia, hypercarbia, bronchospasm, and residual neuromuscular blockade.
- *Cardiovascular instability*: Hypotension, hypertension, arrhythmias, and bleeding.
- *Neurologic issues*: Delayed emergence, agitation, delirium, stroke, and seizure.
- *Pain/nausea*: Require prompt multimodal management.

18.4 Phases of Recovery

18.4.1 Phase I Recovery

- *Focus*: Physiologic stabilization, close monitoring of airway, ventilation, hemodynamics, and neurologic recovery.
- *Monitoring*: American Society of Anesthesiologists (ASA) standards recommend continuous monitoring until the patient regains protective reflexes and stable vital signs.
- *Staffing*: High-intensity, typically 1:1 nursing.

18.4.2 Phase II Recovery

- *Focus*: Preparing patients for discharge to home or ward; emphasis on comfort, oral intake, ambulation, and patient/family education.
- *Setting*: Often occurs in same-day surgery or step-down units with lower intensity of monitoring.
- *Staffing*: Nursing ratios are less intense (e.g., 1:2 to 1:3).

18.5 Discharge Criteria from PACU

Discharge must be systematic, ensuring that the patient is physiologically stable, comfortable, and safe to transition. Two widely used scoring systems include Aldrete and the modified post-anesthesia discharge scoring system (PADSS), which are demonstrated in Tables 18.1 and 18.2, respectively.

Table 18.1 Aldrete score

Parameter	0 Points	1 Point	2 Points
Activity	Cannot move extremities	Moves 2 extremities	Moves 4 extremities voluntarily/on command
Respiration	Apneic	Dyspneic, shallow, or limited	Able to breathe deeply and cough freely
Circulation	BP >50 mmHg different from preop	BP 20–50 mmHg different from preop	BP ±20 mmHg of preop level
Consciousness	Not responding	Arousable on calling	Fully awake
O_2 saturation	<90% even with O_2	Needs O_2 to maintain >90%	>92% on room air

Interpretation: Score ≥9/10 is generally required for PACU discharge

Table 18.2 Modified PADSS

Parameter	0 Points	1 Point	2 Points
Vital signs	Abnormal: >40% of baseline	Abnormal: 20–40% of baseline	Within 20% of baseline
Ambulation	Unable to ambulate	Ambulates with assistance	Ambulates without assistance
Nausea/vomiting	Severe, requires treatment	Moderate, controlled with treatment	Minimal or none
Pain	Severe, uncontrolled	Moderate, controlled with oral meds	Minimal or adequately controlled
Bleeding	Severe, requires intervention	Moderate, requires dressing change	Minimal

Interpretation: Score ≥9/10 is required for safe discharge after ambulatory surgery

18.6 Handoffs in the PACU

Effective communication between anesthesia providers and PACU nurses is critical. Standardized handoff tools (e.g., Situation, Background, Assessment, Recommendation) improve information transfer, reduce errors, and enhance patient safety.

18.7 Systems-Based Aspects

18.7.1 Safety and Monitoring Standards

- ASA mandates monitoring until discharge criteria are met.
- Policies should ensure the continuous availability of trained personnel.

18.7.2 Quality Metrics

PACU performance is often measured by unplanned ICU admissions, re-intubations, unexpected hospitalizations after ambulatory surgery, and patient satisfaction.

18.7.3 Pain and Post Operative Nausea and Vomiting (PONV) Management

- *Pain (see* Chap. 28 *for more information)*: Multimodal strategies combining opioids, NSAIDs, acetaminophen, and regional blocks.
- *PONV (see* Chap. 25 *for more information)*: Prophylaxis guided by risk factors (female sex, nonsmoker, history of motion sickness, and opioid use).

18.8 Common PACU Complications

- *Airway/Respiratory*: Hypoxemia, laryngospasm, and residual blockade.
- *Cardiovascular*: Hypotension, hypertension, arrhythmias, and bleeding.
- *Neurologic*: Delayed emergence, agitation, and delirium.
- *Other*: Hypothermia, shivering, and urinary retention.

18.9 Special Populations

18.9.1 Pediatrics

- Risks: Airway obstruction, laryngospasm, and emergence delirium.

18.9.2 Geriatrics

- Risks: Delirium, prolonged recovery, and hypothermia.

18.9.3 High-Risk Patients

- ASA III/IV, obstructive sleep apnea (OSA), obesity, and cardiac/pulmonary disease → may require extended PACU or ICU stay.

18.10 Conclusion

The PACU is a critical environment bridging the OR and ward, providing vigilant monitoring during one of the most physiologically unstable phases of care. Its structure emphasizes proximity to surgical suites, intensive nursing, and ready access to resuscitation equipment. Assessment follows a systematic airway–breathing–circulation–neurologic–pain framework. Recovery is staged (Phase I stabilization, Phase II preparation for discharge), and validated discharge criteria, such as the Aldrete Score and PADSS, standardize readiness for transfer.

PACU care is multidisciplinary, requiring coordination between anesthesiologists, nurses, surgeons, and internists. For internists, understanding PACU principles clarifies early postoperative complications and informs collaborative care after transfer. Ultimately, the PACU embodies the principles of perioperative medicine: vigilance, safety, structured assessment, and timely intervention.

Key Takeaways

1. The PACU provides structured monitoring and stabilization during the vulnerable immediate post-anesthesia period.
2. Assessment follows a systematic approach: airway, breathing, circulation, neurologic status, and pain.
3. Recovery occurs in phases: Phase I (intensive stabilization) and Phase II (readiness for discharge).
4. Discharge requires meeting validated criteria (Aldrete ≥9 or PADSS ≥9).
5. Effective handoffs, multimodal pain/PONV management, and interdisciplinary collaboration are essential for safe PACU operations.

Suggested Reading

1. Apfelbaum JL, Silverstein JH, Chung FF, et al. Practice guidelines for postanesthetic care. Anesthesiology. 2013;118(2):291–307.
2. Aseni P, Orsenigo S, Storti E, et al. Current concepts of perioperative monitoring in high-risk surgical patients: a review. Patient Saf Surg. 2019;13:32.
3. Aldrete JA. The post-anesthesia recovery score revisited. J Clin Anesth. 1995;7(1):89–91.
4. Chung F, Chan VW, Ong D. A post-anesthetic discharge scoring system for home readiness after ambulatory surgery. J Clin Anesth. 1995;7(6):500–6.
5. Sessler DI. Temperature monitoring and perioperative thermoregulation. Anesthesiology. 2008;109(2):318–38.
6. Monk TG, Weldon BC, Garvan CW, et al. Predictors of cognitive dysfunction after major noncardiac surgery. Anesthesiology. 2008;108(1):18–30.
7. Duffy CC, Lepore G, Bass GA. A systematic review of postoperative care transition interventions: examining the implementation of handoff protocols and checklists. Anesth Analg. 2025. https://doi.org/10.1213/ANE.0000000000007523. Online ahead of print.

19 Postoperative Delirium, Cognitive Dysfunction, Delayed Emergence, and Intraoperative Awareness

19.1 Introduction

Anesthesia and surgery exert profound effects on the central nervous system. Although most patients recover without complication, a subset develops postoperative alterations in consciousness and cognition that may prolong hospitalization, diminish quality of life, and increase mortality. Understanding the distinctions among postoperative delirium, postoperative cognitive dysfunction (POCD), delayed emergence, and intraoperative awareness allows clinicians to identify risk factors, anticipate complications, and intervene early.

19.2 Postoperative Delirium

19.2.1 Definition and Clinical Features

Delirium is an acute disturbance in attention, awareness, and cognition, characterized by a fluctuating course and impaired ability to focus or sustain attention. It typically arises within the first 24–72 h after surgery. Subtypes include hyperactive, hypoactive, and mixed presentations.

19.2.2 Risk Factors

- *Patient factors*: Advanced age, frailty, dementia, sensory impairment, depression, and malnutrition
- *Medical comorbidities*: Cardiovascular disease, renal/hepatic impairment, infection, and metabolic derangements
- *Surgical/anesthetic factors*: Major surgery (e.g., cardiac, orthopedic, and abdominal), blood loss, transfusion, prolonged anesthesia, postoperative pain, opioid, or anticholinergic medications

A. Mirrakhimov, *Anesthesiology Demystified for the Internist*,
https://doi.org/10.1007/978-3-032-16811-5_19

19.2.3 Pathophysiology

Delirium is multifactorial, involving neurotransmitter imbalance (acetylcholine deficiency and dopamine excess), neuroinflammation, oxidative stress, and impaired cerebral autoregulation.

19.2.4 Workup and Diagnosis

- *Clinical diagnosis:* Confusion Assessment Method (CAM) or CAM-Intensive Care Unit (ICU).
- *Exclude reversible causes:* hypoxemia, hypercarbia, hypoglycemia, electrolyte derangements, infection, and medication toxicity
- Imaging or electroencephalogram (EEG) if focal deficits or seizures are suspected

19.2.5 Prevention

- Risk stratification for high-risk patients
- Orientation protocols and cognitive stimulation
- Sleep hygiene, noise reduction, and early mobilization
- Adequate pain control with multimodal strategies, minimizing opioids and anticholinergics
- Avoidance of deep or prolonged sedation in ICU patients (e.g., benzodiazepine-sparing protocols)

19.2.6 Management

- Correct underlying causes.
- Non-pharmacologic strategies (e.g., reorientation, mobilization, and sensory aids).
- Antipsychotics (e.g., haloperidol) for severe agitation threatening safety.
- Dexmedetomidine infusions can reduce delirium incidence in select ICU patients.

19.3 Postoperative Cognitive Dysfunction

19.3.1 Definition and Clinical Features

POCD is a decline in cognitive performance (memory, attention, and executive function) persisting weeks to months after surgery. Unlike delirium, it is insidious, often identified by formal neuropsychological testing rather than acute changes.

19.3.2 Risk Factors

- *Age*: The elderly most vulnerable
- *Baseline cognition*: Dementia and low cognitive reserve
- *Comorbidities*: Atherosclerosis, diabetes, and sleep apnea
- *Surgical*: Major/prolonged procedures and cardiac surgery with cardiopulmonary bypass
- *Anesthetic*: Depth of anesthesia, hypotension, and hypoxemia

19.3.3 Pathophysiology

Likely reflects neuroinflammation, cerebral microemboli (notably in cardiac surgery), hypoperfusion, and interplay with neurodegenerative processes.

19.3.4 Workup and Diagnosis

- Neuropsychological testing before and after surgery (memory, attention, and executive function).
- Rule out delirium, depression, medication effects, and metabolic derangements.

19.3.5 Prevention

- Optimize comorbidities preoperatively.
- Minimize deep anesthesia (processed EEG to avoid burst suppression).
- Early mobilization, physical, and cognitive rehabilitation strategies.

19.3.6 Role of Anesthetic Technique

The influence of anesthetic mode (general vs. regional/neuraxial) on POCD has been extensively studied. Multiple randomized controlled trials and meta-analyses suggest no consistent long-term difference in POCD incidence between general and regional anesthesia. While regional techniques may reduce immediate postoperative delirium risk in some settings, long-term cognitive outcomes appear more influenced by patient age, comorbidities, surgical invasiveness, and perioperative complications rather than anesthetic type alone. Thus, anesthetic mode should be chosen primarily based on surgical requirements and patient comorbidities.

19.3.7 Management

- Supportive care and cognitive rehabilitation.

- Treat reversible contributors (e.g., sleep disturbance, depression, and medications).
- No proven pharmacologic treatment.

19.4 Delayed Emergence

19.4.1 Definition

Failure to regain consciousness within 30–60 minutes after discontinuation of anesthetics.

19.4.2 Causes

1. *Residual drugs*: Potential pharmacologic contributors include inhaled anesthetics, particularly in prolonged cases, where accumulation in adipose and muscle tissue serves as a reservoir for volatile agents and may be exacerbated by ineffective ventilation. Intravenous agents such as propofol, benzodiazepines, and barbiturates. Opioids and neuromuscular blocking agents, especially in the context of inadequate reversal, may further contribute to delayed emergence.
2. *Metabolic*: Hypoglycemia, hypo-/hypernatremia, hypocalcemia, hypothermia, hypoxemia, and hypercarbia.
3. *Neurologic*: Stroke, seizure, raised intracranial pressure (ICP), and anoxic brain injury.
4. *Endocrine*: Severe hypothyroidism and adrenal insufficiency.

19.4.3 Workup

- Review drug history and timing of anesthetic discontinuation.
- Labs: arterial blood gas (ABG), electrolytes, and glucose.
- Neurologic exam ± imaging if focal deficits.

19.4.4 Prevention

- Avoidance of excessive anesthetic dosing
- Using processed EEG or clinical depth monitoring in high-risk cases
- Monitoring neuromuscular blockade and ensuring full reversal
- Maintenance of normothermia and metabolic homeostasis intraoperatively

19.4.5 Management

- Airway support and ventilation until recovery.
- Reverse residual drugs: naloxone (opioids), flumazenil (benzodiazepines), and sugammadex/neostigmine (non-depolarizers).
- Correct metabolic disturbances.
- Neurologic evaluation for persistent unexplained cases.

19.5 Intraoperative Awareness

19.5.1 Definition

Explicit recall of events during general anesthesia. Rare (0.1–0.2%) but associated with post-traumatic stress disorder, anxiety, and litigation.

19.5.2 Risk Factors

- *Patient*: Chronic opioid/benzodiazepine use, substance abuse, and prior awareness.
- *Surgical*: Trauma, obstetric, and cardiac surgery patients are at increased risk because they often cannot hemodynamically tolerate full anesthetic doses. In cardiac surgery, anesthetic delivery typically occurs through the cardiopulmonary bypass circuit, where dosing may be inadequate due to variability in administration and the perfusionist's limited anesthesia agents knowledge and expertise.
- *Anesthetic*: Inadequate dosing, equipment malfunction, total intravenous anesthesia (TIVA) without processed EEG, and neuromuscular blockade masking movement.

19.5.3 Pathophysiology

Occurs when anesthetic depth is insufficient relative to surgical stimulation, especially if hemodynamic constraints limit anesthetic dosing.

19.5.4 Prevention

- Identify high-risk patients preoperatively.
- Maintain adequate anesthetic depth (end-tidal volatile concentration ≥0.7–1.0 MAC when feasible).
- Use processed EEG (e.g., bispectral index (BIS)) during TIVA.
- Avoid unnecessary neuromuscular blockade without ensuring adequate depth.
- Vigilant equipment checks.

19.5.5 Workup and Detection

- Structured postoperative interview.
- Differentiate from dreams or delirium.

19.5.6 Management

- Immediate intraoperative: Deepen anesthesia and administer amnestic agents (benzodiazepine).
- Postoperative: Acknowledge, disclose, provide psychological support, and psychiatric referral if needed.

19.6 Conclusion

Postoperative delirium, POCD, delayed emergence, and intraoperative awareness are important perioperative complications of consciousness and cognition. Delirium is acute and fluctuating, POCD is insidious and prolonged, delayed emergence reflects failure to awaken promptly, and intraoperative awareness involves explicit recall. Prevention strategies ranging from multimodal analgesia and orientation protocols to anesthetic depth monitoring are central.

Mode of anesthesia (general vs. regional) does not appear to significantly alter long-term POCD risk, though it may influence delirium incidence in specific populations. Internists and anesthesiologists must collaborate to anticipate risks, ensure systematic workups, and provide patient-centered management. These conditions underscore that anesthesia extends beyond the intraoperative period, with implications for both short- and long-term outcomes.

Key Takeaways

1. *Postoperative delirium* is common and often preventable with orientation, mobilization, and opioid-sparing analgesia.
2. *POCD* persists for weeks to months; risk depends more on age, comorbidities, and surgical stress than anesthetic technique.
3. *Delayed emergence* requires systematic evaluation for drug, metabolic, and neurologic causes; prevention involves careful titration and monitoring.
4. *Intraoperative awareness* is rare but devastating; prevention includes anesthetic depth monitoring and cautious use of neuromuscular blockade.
5. Prevention strategies—patient optimization, intraoperative vigilance, and structured discharge evaluation—are as crucial as treatment for these neurologic complications.

Suggested Reading

1. Inouye SK, Westendorp RGJ, Saczynski JS. Delirium in elderly people. Lancet. 2014;383(9920):911–22.
2. Radtke FM, Franck M, Lendner J, et al. Monitoring depth of anaesthesia in a randomized trial decreases the rate of postoperative delirium but not postoperative cognitive dysfunction. Br J Anaesth. 2013;110(Suppl 1):i98–105.
3. Bilotta F, Lauretta MP, Borozdina A, et al. Postoperative delirium: risk factors, diagnosis and perioperative care. Minerva Anestesiol. 2013;79(9):1066–76.
4. Rundshagen I. Postoperative cognitive dysfunction. Dtsch Arztebl Int. 2014;111(8):119–25.
5. Cascella M, Bimonte S, Di Napoli R. Delayed emergence from anesthesia: what we know and how we act. Local Reg Anesth. 2020;13:195–206.
6. Bruchas RR, Kent CD, Wilson HD, et al. Anesthesia awareness: narrative review of psychological sequelae, treatment, and incidence. J Clin Psychol Med Settings. 2011;18(3):257–67.
7. Messina AG, Wang M, Ward MJ, et al. Anaesthetic interventions for prevention of awareness during surgery. Cochrane Database Syst Rev. 2016;10(10):CD007272.
8. Chen Q, Peng S, Luo W, et al. Preventive strategies for reducing intraoperative awareness due to errors in anesthetic drug delivery systems: a narrative review. Front Pharmacol. 2025;16:1566185.

Postoperative Cardiac Complications: Myocardial Infarction, Arrhythmias, Heart Failure, and Tamponade

20

20.1 Introduction

Despite advances in perioperative care, cardiovascular complications remain among the most feared postoperative events. Their incidence varies with surgical complexity, patient comorbidity, and perioperative optimization, but they disproportionately contribute to morbidity, mortality, and cost. Most patients who develop postoperative cardiac complications have a pre-existing history of heart disease.

The four entities addressed here, including myocardial infarction (MI), arrhythmias, heart failure, and tamponade, highlight the spectrum of acute postoperative cardiac issues. They differ in pathophysiology and prognosis, but all demand prompt recognition, systematic evaluation, and early involvement of cardiology and cardiac surgery teams to guide definitive therapy.

20.2 Postoperative MI

20.2.1 Epidemiology and Etiology

Perioperative MI (PMI) occurs in 2–6% of patients undergoing major non-cardiac surgery, with a higher incidence after vascular and thoracic procedures. Mechanisms include:

- Type I (plaque rupture and thrombosis)
- Type II (supply-demand mismatch), far more common in the perioperative setting

20.2.2 Presentation in the Postoperative Patient

- *Symptoms are often absent*: Analgesia, sedation, or surgical pain can mask ischemic chest pain.

A. Mirrakhimov, *Anesthesiology Demystified for the Internist*,
https://doi.org/10.1007/978-3-032-16811-5_20

- *Subtle signs*: Hypotension, tachycardia, arrhythmia, dyspnea, or unexpected decline in functional status.
- *Biomarkers*: Troponin elevations are common but require correlation with electrocardiogram (ECG) or imaging.
- *ECG*: ST-segment changes can be nonspecific and easily overlooked.

20.2.3 Diagnosis

- High-risk patients often undergo routine troponin surveillance.
- Echocardiography may reveal new wall motion abnormalities.
- Coronary angiography is considered for unstable or high-risk anatomy.

20.2.4 Management Nuances

In all cases of suspected PMI, cardiology should be urgently consulted to guide diagnostic workup and decisions about revascularization, anticoagulation, and dual antiplatelet therapy (DAPT) in the context of surgical bleeding risk. It is also essential to notify the primary surgical or procedural team, given the potential risk and morbidity associated with bleeding at the surgical site (e.g., in neurosurgical patients).

- *Antiplatelet therapy*: Aspirin should be continued; initiation of DAPT requires careful assessment of bleeding risk in consultation with cardiology and the primary surgical team.
- *Anticoagulation*: Heparinization must be balanced with surgical hemostasis.
- *Revascularization*: Percutaneous coronary intervention (PCI) may be lifesaving, but the surgical context complicates timing; urgent cardiology input is essential.
- *Medical therapy*: Beta-blockers, statins, and ACE inhibitors should be optimized.

20.3 Postoperative Arrhythmias

20.3.1 Epidemiology and Etiology

Arrhythmias, especially atrial fibrillation (AF), are common postoperatively. Incidence ranges from 10–40% after thoracic or cardiac surgery, but also occurs after non-cardiac procedures. Triggers include catecholamine surge, electrolyte imbalance, hypoxemia, acidosis, fluid shifts, and beta-blocker withdrawal.

20.3.2 Types and Presentations

- *Atrial fibrillation (AF)/atrial flutter*: Often asymptomatic but may destabilize hemodynamics
- *Ventricular arrhythmias*: Frequently secondary to ischemia or electrolyte imbalance
- *Bradyarrhythmias*: From ischemia, conduction disease, or vagal stimulation

20.3.3 Workup

- ECG and continuous telemetry
- Electrolytes, arterial blood gas (ABG), and thyroid testing as indicated
- Troponin if ischemia suspected

20.3.4 Management Nuances

- *Rate control*: Beta-blockers or calcium channel blockers are preferred; amiodarone may be used if refractory, though it carries a small risk of cardioversion to sinus rhythm and potential embolization in the presence of an in situ cardiac thrombus, particularly in long-standing AF.
- *Rhythm control*: Reserved for unstable patients or recurrent symptomatic AF.
- *Anticoagulation*: Stroke prevention must be individualized, given high bleeding risk; cardiology and primary surgical team collaboration is crucial.
- *Ventricular arrhythmias*: Management includes supportive care, correction of electrolyte abnormalities, adherence to advanced cardiovascular life support (ACLS) protocols for hemodynamically unstable ventricular rhythms, and evaluation for underlying ischemia or metabolic disturbances.
- *Bradyarrhythmias*: Atropine, dopamine, epinephrine, and pacing if severe.

20.3.5 Prevention

- Correct electrolytes, optimize oxygenation, and continue perioperative beta-blockers.

20.3.6 Key Point

Cardiology consultation is invaluable for risk stratification, anticoagulation timing, and long-term arrhythmia management strategies.

20.4 Postoperative Heart Failure

20.4.1 Epidemiology and Etiology

Postoperative heart failure exacerbation is common, particularly in patients with prior ventricular dysfunction. Causes include fluid overload, transfusion-associated circulatory overload, ischemia, and arrhythmias.

20.4.2 Presentation in the Postoperative Patient

- Symptoms may be subtle (dyspnea masked by sedation).
- Signs: hypoxemia, rales, jugular venous distention, and body edema.
- Chest x-ray (CXR): pulmonary edema; echocardiography to assess ventricular function and presence of valvular heart disease.

20.4.3 Management Nuances

- *Diuresis*: Loop diuretics first line.
- *Oxygenation*: Non-invasive ventilation, such as bilevel positive airway pressure (BiPAP), may avert intubation in some patients.
- *Inotropes*: Dobutamine and milrinone for cardiogenic shock.
- *Afterload reduction*: Used carefully due to perioperative hypotension risk.
- *Fluids*: Restrict further overload; tailor based on hemodynamics.

20.4.4 Prevention

- Conservative fluid management intra- and postoperatively in patients at risk
- Continuation of chronic HF medications
- Preoperative optimization for known HF patients

Early cardiology involvement is essential for tailoring diuretic regimens, optimizing inotropes/vasodilators, and planning advanced therapies if decompensation persists.

20.5 Postoperative Cardiac Tamponade

20.5.1 Epidemiology and Etiology

Tamponade is rare but life-threatening, usually after cardiac/thoracic surgery, interventional cardiology, and electrophysiology procedures (e.g., left atrial appendage occlusion, AF ablation, and interventional cardiology valve procedures such as edge-to-edge mitral valve repair).

20.5.2 Pathophysiology

Rapid pericardial fluid accumulation restricts diastolic filling → obstructive shock.

20.5.3 Presentation in the Postoperative Patient

- Classic Beck triad (hypotension, muffled heart sounds, jugular venous distention) is often absent.
- Signs: hypotension, tachycardia, elevated central venous pressure (CVP), and oliguria.
- Echocardiography confirms the diagnosis.

20.5.4 Management Nuances

- *Definitive treatment*: Surgical re-exploration (especially after cardiac surgery).
- *Percutaneous drainage*: Pericardiocentesis has a limited role in postcardiac surgery clotted hemopericardium, for which immediate cardiac surgery notification is essential. However, pericardiocentesis remains central in managing tamponade related to interventional cardiology or electrophysiology procedures.
- *Supportive care*: Vasopressors and intravenous fluid administration.

20.6 Conclusion

Postoperative cardiac complications such as MI, arrhythmias, heart failure, and tamponade are common, high-impact conditions that require vigilance and rapid response. Their presentations are often atypical due to analgesia, sedation, or surgical context, and their management must balance cardiology guidelines with surgical constraints such as bleeding risk and wound healing.

A consistent theme is that early and close collaboration with cardiology and, when indicated, cardiac surgery teams is paramount. Interdisciplinary care ensures that treatment is not only guideline-driven but also safe and patient-centered in the delicate postoperative context.

Key Takeaways

1. MI is often silent postoperatively; cardiology should be consulted urgently to guide diagnosis and treatment.
2. Arrhythmias are common; stroke prevention in patients with atrial fibrillation and long-term management require cardiology input, especially for anticoagulation timing.

3. Heart failure management must balance diuresis and organ perfusion.
4. Cardiac tamponade is an emergency; immediate cardiology or cardiac surgery consultation is critical.
5. Across all complications, early involvement of cardiology and cardiac surgery teams improves outcomes and should be standard practice.

Suggested Reading

1. Devereaux PJ, Biccard BM, Sigamani A, et al. Association of postoperative high-sensitivity troponin levels with myocardial injury and 30-day mortality among patients undergoing non-cardiac surgery. JAMA. 2017;317(16):1642–51.
2. Ruetzler K, Smilowitz NR, Berger JS, et al. Diagnosis and management of patients with myocardial injury after noncardiac surgery: a scientific statement from the American Heart Association. Circulation. 2021;144(19):e287–305.
3. Rostagno C, Craighero A. Postoperative myocardial infarction after non-cardiac surgery: an update. J Clin Med. 2024;13(5):1473.
4. Peretto G, Durante A, Limite LR, et al. Postoperative arrhythmias after cardiac surgery: incidence, risk factors, and therapeutic management. Cardiol Res Pract. 2014;2014:615987.
5. Shah S, Chahil V, Battisha A, et al. Postoperative atrial fibrillation: a review. Biomedicines. 2024;12(9):1968.
6. Lerman BJ, Popat RA, Assimes TL, et al. Association between heart failure and postoperative mortality among patients undergoing ambulatory noncardiac surgery. JAMA Surg. 2019;154(10):907–14.
7. Carmona P, Mateo E, Casanovas I, et al. Management of cardiac tamponade after cardiac surgery. J Cardiothorac Vasc Anesth. 2012;26(2):302–11.
8. Russo CM, Harrison ME, Harry NM, et al. Intraoperative acute cardiac tamponade as a result of intracardiac perforation requiring emergency continuous pericardiocentesis and open sternotomy: a case report and literature review of a rare but fatal complication. Cureus. 2024;16(2):e54701.
9. Adamczyk M, Wasilewski J, Niedziela J, et al. Pericardial tamponade as a complication of invasive cardiac procedures: a review of the literature. Postepy Kardiol Interwencyjnej. 2019;15(4):394–403.
10. Madhivathanan PR, Corredor C, Smith A. Perioperative implications of pericardial effusions and cardiac tamponade. BJA Educ. 2020;20(7):226–34.

Postoperative Pulmonary Complications: Hypoventilation, Atelectasis, Pneumonia, Pulmonary Embolism, and Acute Respiratory Distress Syndrome

21

21.1 Introduction

Respiratory complications are among the most common adverse outcomes after surgery and anesthesia, often rivaling cardiac complications in incidence and negative impact on outcomes. Their prevention and management require an understanding of the interaction of patient risk factors, surgical stresses, and anesthetic influences on the respiratory system.

Unlike medical respiratory disease, postoperative pulmonary complications (PPCs) are frequently multifactorial, arising from a combination of pre-existing comorbidities, intraoperative factors (e.g., mechanical ventilation, positioning, anesthetic agents, etc.), and postoperative challenges (e.g., pain, sedation, and immobility). Early detection is often challenging, as symptoms such as dyspnea or chest pain may be masked by analgesia, sedation, or limited mobility.

21.2 Hypoventilation

21.2.1 Etiology and Risk Factors

Hypoventilation in the postoperative period results from inadequate alveolar ventilation relative to metabolic demand. Causes include the following:

- *Pre-existing disorders*
  - *Obstructive sleep apnea (OSA)*: Upper airway collapse worsened by sedatives, opioids, and potential residual neuromuscular block.
  - *Obesity hypoventilation syndrome (OHS)*: Reduced ventilatory drive and restrictive pulmonary mechanics.
- *Residual anesthetic and sedative effects*
  - Propofol, benzodiazepines, and opioids suppress respiratory drive.

A. Mirrakhimov, *Anesthesiology Demystified for the Internist*,
https://doi.org/10.1007/978-3-032-16811-5_21

- *Residual neuromuscular blockade*
  - Incomplete reversal leads to muscle weakness, impaired airway protection, and shallow ventilation.
- *Central nervous system pathology*
  - Stroke, seizure, and intracranial hemorrhage can depress the central respiratory drive.
- *Metabolic causes*
  - Hypoglycemia (critical to exclude in patients with altered mental status).
  - Severe electrolyte disturbances (e.g., hypokalemia, hyponatremia, and hypocalcemia).
  - Metabolic acidosis leading to fatigue of ventilatory muscles.
- *Pain-related hypoventilation*
  - Splinting after thoracic or abdominal surgery.
- *Airway obstruction*
  - Macroglossia, edema, poor positioning, or laryngospasm.

21.2.2 Clinical Presentation

- Bradypnea or shallow breathing
- Hypoxemia and hypercarbia on monitoring
- Altered consciousness, somnolence, or agitation
- In severe cases: apnea or cardiopulmonary arrest

21.2.3 Management

- Immediate airway assessment and support.
- Rule out hypoglycemia with point-of-care glucose measurement.
- Arterial blood gas for hypercarbia, metabolic acidosis, and electrolyte abnormalities.
- Reversal agents: naloxone for opioids, flumazenil for benzodiazepines, and sugammadex or neostigmine for residual blockade.
- Noninvasive ventilation is appropriate for OSA/OHS or mild hypoventilation in patients without altered mental status or aspiration risk. It should be avoided in select surgical populations, such as after transsphenoidal pituitary surgery (risk of pneumocephalus) or esophagectomy (risk of gastrointestinal insufflation and impaired anastomotic healing), in whom endotracheal intubation is indicated if respiratory distress develops.
- Intubation and controlled ventilation if refractory.

21.2.4 Prevention

- Preoperative OSA screening
- Cautious opioid and sedative dosing, multimodal analgesia
- Quantitative neuromuscular monitoring with full reversal
- Frequent glucose checks in diabetics or after prolonged surgery

21.3 Atelectasis

21.3.1 Etiology

Atelectasis is nearly universal after general anesthesia, due to absorption of alveolar gas, compression, or surfactant dysfunction. Risk factors include obesity, long surgical procedures, supine position, and poor inspiratory effort.

21.3.2 Clinical Presentation

- Hypoxemia, diminished breath sounds, and dullness to percussion
- Radiograph or ultrasound: areas of collapse, often in dependent lung zones

21.3.3 Management

- Incentive spirometry, early mobilization, and deep breathing
- Continuous positive airway pressure (CPAP) or noninvasive ventilation for high-risk patients
- Analgesia to allow deep breathing and coughing (e.g., epidural for pain control after thoracotomy)

21.3.4 Prevention

- Intraoperative positive end expiratory pressure (PEEP) and recruitment maneuvers
- Avoidance of unnecessary high FiO_2

21.4 Pneumonia and Aspiration

21.4.1 Etiology

- *Pneumonia*: Develops from impaired clearance, atelectasis, aspiration, or prolonged mechanical ventilation.
- *Aspiration pneumonitis*: Chemical injury from gastric contents; may evolve into pneumonia.

21.4.2 Risk Factors

- Residual sedation or opioids → impaired airway reflexes.
- Difficult intubation, reflux, and ileus.
- Age, frailty, and neuromuscular disease.

21.4.3 Clinical Presentation

- Fever, leukocytosis, hypoxemia, and new infiltrates.
- Aspiration is often sudden with hypoxemia and bronchospasm.

21.4.4 Management

- *Aspiration pneumonitis*: Supportive care; antibiotics only if infection suspected >48 h.
- *Pneumonia*: Empiric antibiotics guided by hospital versus community context, then de-escalate by cultures.
- Pulmonary toilet and chest physiotherapy.

21.4.5 Prevention

- Strict nil per os (nothing by mouth) (NPO) guidelines.
- Rapid sequence induction in patients at high risk
- Cuffed endotracheal tube (ETT) instead of laryngeal mask airway (LMA) for patients with high aspiration risk.
- Awake extubation with intact reflexes.
- Elevate the head of bed.

21.5 Pulmonary Embolism (PE)

21.5.1 Etiology and Risk Factors

Major risk factors include orthopedic, pelvic, and cancer surgery, previous venous thromboembolic event.

21.5.2 Clinical Presentation

- Dyspnea, tachycardia, hypoxemia, and hypotension
- Unexplained hypoxemia in post operative care unit (PACU) or ward

21.5.3 Diagnosis

- CT pulmonary angiography.
- Echocardiography can be supportive for clinically significant PE but lacks specificity.
- D-dimer is of limited role in the postoperative period due to poor specificity and almost universal elevation.

21.5.4 Management

- Anticoagulation if bleeding risk is acceptable.
- Inferior vena cava (IVC) filter if anticoagulation is contraindicated.
- Thrombolysis, embolectomy (e.g., minimally invasive or surgical), and veno-arterial extracorporeal membrane oxygenation (ECMO) support for massive PE.

21.5.5 Prevention

- LMWH or heparin prophylaxis
- Compression devices and early ambulation

21.6 Acute Respiratory Distress Syndrome (ARDS)

21.6.1 Etiology

Triggers include sepsis, aspiration, trauma, thoracic surgery, and blood product transfusion, such as transfusion-related acute lung injury.

21.6.2 Clinical Presentation

- Severe hypoxemia refractory to supplemental O_2 is indicative of a shunt.
- Bilateral infiltrates on imaging.

21.6.3 Management

The management is similar to ARDS in non-surgical patients.

- Lung-protective ventilation: low tidal volume and PEEP titration
- Prone positioning for severe ARDS
- Restrictive fluids
- ECMO in refractory centers

21.6.4 Prevention

- Judicious transfusion and fluid management
- Prevent aspiration and sepsis

21.7 Negative Pressure Pulmonary Edema

21.7.1 Etiology

Occurs following acute upper airway obstruction, most commonly laryngospasm, when forceful inspiratory efforts against a closed glottis generate markedly negative intrathoracic pressure, leading to pulmonary capillary stress failure and fluid transudation into the alveoli.

21.7.2 Clinical Presentation

- Sudden hypoxemia, pink frothy sputum, and distress after an obstruction episode.

21.7.3 Management

- Relieves airway obstruction and provides supplemental oxygen.
- Apply CPAP or intubate and ventilate with PEEP.
- Supportive care. Most cases will resolve within 24–48 h.
- Veno-venous ECMO may be considered in refractory cases, offering a generally favorable prognosis when instituted early prior to the onset of hypoxemic cerebral injury.

21.7.4 Prevention

- Smooth extubation with airway reflexes intact
- Vigilance for laryngospasm

21.8 Conclusion

PPCs are common and often multifactorial. Hypoventilation may result from residual sedation, incomplete reversal of neuromuscular blockade, central nervous system events, airway obstruction, or metabolic disturbances such as hypoglycemia and electrolyte abnormalities—all of which should be promptly excluded. Atelectasis is nearly universal after general anesthesia, while pneumonia and aspiration remain major sources of morbidity, particularly in high-risk patients. PE, though preventable, continues to be a major cause of postoperative morbidity and mortality, and ARDS represents severe inflammatory lung injury. Negative pressure pulmonary edema, though uncommon, exemplifies airway-related complications unique to the anesthetic setting.

Prevention is through meticulous intraoperative ventilatory management, judicious fluid administration, multimodal analgesia, venous thromboembolism prophylaxis, and early mobilization—remains the most effective strategy. Close collaboration among anesthesiology, surgery, medicine, and critical care teams is essential for early recognition and timely intervention.

Key Takeaways

1. Hypoventilation requires systematic evaluation, including ruling out metabolic causes such as hypoglycemia and electrolyte derangements.
2. Atelectasis is nearly universal under general anesthesia and contributes to many PPCs; prevention involves mobilization, pain control, and lung expansion maneuvers.
3. Pneumonia and aspiration are major causes of morbidity; prevention depends on airway protection, pulmonary hygiene, and infection control.
4. PE is a preventable but often deadly complication; anticoagulant prophylaxis and ambulation are key.
5. ARDS and negative pressure pulmonary edema highlight inflammatory and airway-related risks requiring early recognition and lung-protective strategies.

Suggested Readings

1. Lusquinhos J, Tavares M, Abelha F. Postoperative pulmonary complications and perioperative strategies: a systematic review. Cureus. 2023;15(5):e38786.
2. Miskovic A, Lumb AB. Postoperative pulmonary complications. Br J Anaesth. 2017;118(3):317–34.
3. Neto AS, Schultz MJ, Gama de Abreu M. Intraoperative ventilation strategies to prevent postoperative pulmonary complications: systematic review, meta-analysis, and trial sequential analysis. Best Pract Res Clin Anaesthesiol. 2015;29(3):331–40.
4. Bhattacharya M, Kallet RH, Ware LB, et al. Negative-pressure pulmonary edema. Chest. 2016;150(4):927–33.
5. Porres-Aguilar M, Rivera-Lebron BN, Anaya-Ayala JE, et al. Perioperative acute pulmonary embolism: a concise review with emphasis on multidisciplinary approach. Int J Angiol. 2020;29(3):183–8.
6. Cormican D, Morkos MS, Winter D, et al. Acute perioperative pulmonary embolism-management strategies and outcomes. J Cardiothorac Vasc Anesth. 2020;34(7):1972–84.
7. Sanfilippo F, Palumbo GJ, Bignami E, et al. Acute respiratory distress syndrome in the perioperative period of cardiac surgery: predictors, diagnosis, prognosis, management options, and future directions. J Cardiothorac Vasc Anesth. 2022;36(4):1169–79.
8. Semple JW, Rebetz J, Kapur R. Transfusion-associated circulatory overload and transfusion-related acute lung injury. Blood. 2019;133(17):1840–53.

Postoperative Renal Complications and Acute Kidney Injury

22

22.1 Introduction

Postoperative renal complications are common and clinically significant, particularly in high-risk surgical populations such as those undergoing cardiac, vascular, liver, or major abdominal surgery. Acute kidney injury (AKI) is the most prevalent complication, ranging in incidence from 5% to 30% depending on the patient population and the surgical context. Even mild forms of AKI are associated with adverse outcomes, including increased in-hospital mortality, higher rates of chronic kidney disease (CKD) progression, and long-term cardiovascular morbidity. For anesthesiologists and perioperative clinicians, understanding the mechanisms and modifiable contributors to AKI is essential for prevention and timely management.

22.2 Epidemiology and Clinical Significance

AKI is diagnosed in the postoperative setting using consensus criteria such as Kidney Disease: Improving Global Outcomes (KDIGO). Definitions include an increase in serum creatinine by ≥0.3 mg/dL within 48 h, an increase to ≥1.5 times baseline within 7 days, or urine output <0.5 mL/kg/hour for 6 hours. Incidence varies by surgical population.

Approximate incidence of AKI in different surgical populations:

- *General surgery*: 1–7%
- *Cardiac surgery*: 20–30%
- *Liver transplantation*: up to 50%
- *Major vascular surgery*: 15–20%

Mortality among patients who develop postoperative AKI may be two- to five-fold higher compared to those without AKI. Furthermore, postoperative AKI is a strong predictor of long-term CKD and dialysis dependence.

A. Mirrakhimov, *Anesthesiology Demystified for the Internist*,
https://doi.org/10.1007/978-3-032-16811-5_22

22.3 Pathophysiology

AKI is usually multifactorial and is classically broken down into prerenal, intrinsic, and postrenal mechanisms:

1. *Prerenal*: Hypovolemia, hypotension, systemic vasodilation, increased intra-abdominal pressure, or impaired autoregulation (particularly in elderly or hypertensive patients)
2. *Intrinsic*: Ischemia–reperfusion injury, nephrotoxic medications (e.g., aminoglycosides, radiocontrast, non steroidal anti inflammatory drugs (NSAIDs), etc.), sepsis-associated acute tubular injury, and pigment nephropathy from hemolysis or rhabdomyolysis
3. *Postrenal*: Rare but may occur from ureteral obstruction following pelvic surgery or from bladder outlet obstruction

At a cellular level, perioperative AKI is characterized by endothelial dysfunction, tubular epithelial injury, mitochondrial dysfunction, and dysregulated inflammatory and immune responses.

22.4 Surgery-Specific Mechanisms of AKI

While many mechanisms of perioperative AKI are shared across surgical populations, certain procedures introduce unique risks that merit specific attention.

22.4.1 Embolic Phenomena

Renal embolism during surgery can contribute to postoperative AKI. Manipulation of the aorta in cardiac or major vascular surgery may dislodge atheromatous plaques or thrombotic debris. These emboli can occlude renal arteries or arterioles. Intraoperative risk factors include aortic cross-clamping, cannulation sites, and endovascular stent deployment. Embolic injury often coexists with ischemia–reperfusion and hemodynamic insults, compounding renal damage. Clinically, atheroembolic AKI may be delayed and is sometimes accompanied by livedo reticularis, eosinophilia, or "blue toe" syndrome.

22.4.2 Non-pulsatile Flow During Cardiopulmonary Bypass

Cardiopulmonary bypass (CPB) exposes the kidney to non-physiologic, non-pulsatile flow, systemic inflammatory activation, and hemolysis. The absence of pulsatility can reduce renal perfusion efficiency, impair autoregulation, and contribute to microcirculatory dysfunction. Prolonged CPB time and deep hypothermia further increase susceptibility to ischemia–reperfusion injury. Hemodilution, systemic inflammation, and microemboli are synergistic contributors in this setting.

22.4.3 Surgery-Specific Considerations

- *Cardiac Surgery*:
  AKI incidence is highest in this population due to a combination of CPB-associated insults, embolization, systemic inflammatory response, and low cardiac output syndrome. Off-pump coronary artery bypass grafting (CABG) may reduce AKI in selected patients, though data are mixed.
- *Aortic and Major Vascular Surgery*:
  Aortic cross-clamping can reduce renal blood flow, particularly during suprarenal clamping. Ischemia–reperfusion injury upon unclamping leads to oxidative stress and tubular damage. Embolic events are also common in this setting.
- *Liver Transplantation*:
  Mechanisms include massive blood loss, reperfusion syndrome (abrupt hemodynamic shifts, cytokine release, and inflammatory response), and exposure to nephrotoxic immunosuppressants in the perioperative period.
- *Abdominal Surgery*:
  Increased intra-abdominal pressure from pneumoperitoneum or abdominal compartment syndrome reduces renal perfusion, causing prerenal AKI that may progress to intrinsic damage if uncorrected.
- *Orthopedic Surgery*:
  Fat embolism syndrome and rhabdomyolysis (particularly after prolonged immobilization or compartment syndrome) are unique contributors.

22.5 Risk Factors

22.5.1 Patient-Related

- Advanced age
- Preexisting CKD or reduced estimated glomerular filtration rate (eGFR)
- Diabetes mellitus
- Hypertension
- Heart failure
- Liver disease
- Anemia or hypoalbuminemia

22.5.2 Surgery-Related

- CPB (prolonged bypass and cross-clamp times, low cardiac output)
- Major vascular surgery (aortic cross-clamping, ischemia–reperfusion)
- Orthotopic liver transplantation
- Procedures associated with major blood loss
- Abdominal surgery with raised intra-abdominal pressure

22.5.3 Perioperative/Anesthetic Factors

- Hypotension, especially prolonged mean arterial pressure <65 mmHg
- Excessive fluid administration, causing venous congestion
- Use of nephrotoxic medications (aminoglycosides, amphotericin, calcineurin inhibitors, and high-dose NSAIDs)
- Radiocontrast exposure

22.6 Clinical Presentation

Postoperative AKI is frequently asymptomatic in the early stages. Laboratory findings—serum creatinine rise or oliguria—are often the only indicators. Severe cases may present with:

- Fluid overload and pulmonary edema
- Hyperkalemia
- Metabolic acidosis
- Uremic symptoms (rare in the immediate perioperative period)

22.7 Diagnosis

22.7.1 Laboratory

- Serum creatinine is the principal diagnostic marker; however, its elevation typically lags behind clinical manifestations.
- *Urine output*: Sensitive but influenced by fluids and diuretics.

22.7.2 Imaging

- Renal ultrasound to rule out obstructive uropathy.

22.7.3 Classification

- KDIGO staging is most widely used and correlates with prognosis.

22.8 Prevention Strategies

Preventing perioperative AKI is a primary focus for anesthesiologists. Strategies include the following:

22.8.1 Hemodynamic Optimization

- Maintain mean arterial pressure ≥65 mmHg, with potentially higher targets for patients with chronic hypertension.
- Use of goal-directed therapy with dynamic fluid responsiveness indices.
- Avoidance of sustained hypotension during induction and maintenance.

22.8.2 Fluid Management

- Avoid both hypovolemia and fluid overload.
- Balanced crystalloids (e.g., Plasma-Lyte and Ringer's lactate) are preferred over chloride-rich solutions.
- Avoid hydroxyethyl starch due to the risk of nephrotoxicity.

22.8.3 Pharmacologic Considerations

- Avoid nephrotoxic drugs when possible.
- Avoid the use of NSAIDs in high-risk patients.
- Evidence does not support prophylactic low-dose dopamine or fenoldopam.
- Statins, N-acetylcysteine, and remote ischemic preconditioning show mixed or limited benefit.

22.8.4 Specific Populations

- *Cardiac surgery*: Optimize CPB techniques (e.g. increase CPB flows), minimize hemodilution, and consider off-pump CABG in selected patients, though its benefit remains uncertain due to the risk of profound intraoperative hypotension. While pulsatile flow during off-pump CABG may theoretically confer renal protection, potential hemodynamic instability during the procedure can offset these advantages.
- *Liver transplantation*: Vigilant volume and hemodynamic management, avoidance of excessive transfusion and volume administration.
- *Contrast-associated AKI*: Use the lowest possible dose, iso-osmolar contrast agents, and adequate pre- and post-hydration.

22.9 Management

22.9.1 Supportive Care

- Optimize volume status and perfusion.
- Correct electrolyte disturbances.
- Treat sepsis aggressively.
- Avoid further nephrotoxin exposure.

22.9.2 Diuretics

- Loop diuretics are not therapeutic for AKI but may be used for cases of volume overload.

22.9.3 Renal Replacement Therapy (RRT)

- Indications: Refractory hyperkalemia, metabolic acidosis, fluid overload, and uremic complications.
- Modalities: Intermittent hemodialysis, continuous RRT, or hybrid approaches depending on hemodynamic stability.

22.9.4 Long-Term Implications

Patients with postoperative AKI require close follow-up, as even partial recovery carries increased risk of progression to CKD and cardiovascular events. Early nephrology consultation improves outcomes.

22.10 Conclusion

Postoperative renal complications, particularly AKI, are common, multifactorial, and associated with significant morbidity and mortality. Preventive strategies emphasizing hemodynamic optimization, fluid stewardship, and avoidance of nephrotoxins are the cornerstone of management. Once AKI develops, supportive care and timely initiation of RRT when indicated are key. For anesthesiologists, recognizing risk factors and proactively applying evidence-based strategies can reduce the burden of postoperative AKI and improve patient outcomes.

Key Takeaways

1. *Postoperative AKI is common and multifactorial*, resulting from hemodynamic instability, nephrotoxin exposure, and systemic inflammation, with incidence varying by surgical type.
2. *Surgery-specific mechanisms are major contributors*: Embolization of aortic plaques in vascular and cardiac surgery, non-pulsatile flow and microemboli during CPB, ischemia–reperfusion with aortic cross-clamping, reperfusion syndrome in liver transplantation, and fat embolism or rhabdomyolysis in orthopedic surgery.
3. *Prevention is more effective than treatment*, centering on maintaining renal perfusion pressure, judicious fluid management, and minimizing exposure to nephrotoxins and contrast.

4. *Management of established AKI is supportive*, focusing on hemodynamic optimization, correction of electrolyte disturbances, and initiation of RRT when indicated.
5. *Anesthesiologists play a pivotal role* by recognizing patient- and surgery-specific risk factors, applying evidence-based preventive measures intraoperatively, and ensuring close postoperative monitoring in high-risk populations.

Suggested Reading

1. Ostermann M, Lumlertgul N, Jeong R, et al. Acute kidney injury. Lancet. 2025;405(10474):241–56.
2. Meersch M, Schmidt C, Zarbock A. Perioperative acute kidney injury: an under-recognized problem. Anesth Analg. 2017;125(4):1223–32.
3. Douville NJ, Mathis M, Kheterpal S, et al. Perioperative acute kidney injury: diagnosis, prediction, prevention, and treatment. Anesthesiology. 2024;142(1):180–201.
4. Cheruku SR, Raphael J, Neyra JA, et al. Acute kidney injury after cardiac surgery: prediction, prevention, and management. Anesthesiology. 2023;139(6):880–98.
5. Scurt FG, Bose K, Mertens PR, et al. Cardiac surgery-associated acute kidney injury. Kidney360. 2024;5(6):909–26.
6. Rasmussen SB, Boyko Y, Ranucci M, et al. Cardiac surgery-associated acute kidney injury - a narrative review. Perfusion. 2024;39(8):1516–30.
7. Hobson CE, Yavas S, Segal MS, et al. Acute kidney injury is associated with increased long-term mortality after cardiothoracic surgery. Circulation. 2009;119(18):2444–53.
8. O'Connor ME, Kirwan CJ, Pearse RM, et al. Incidence and associations of acute kidney injury after major abdominal surgery. Intensive Care Med. 2016;42(4):521–30.
9. Prowle JR, Forni LG, Bell M, et al. Postoperative acute kidney injury in adult non-cardiac surgery: joint consensus report of the Acute Disease Quality Initiative and PeriOperative Quality Initiative. Nat Rev Nephrol. 2021;17(9):605–18.

Postoperative Gastrointestinal and Hepatic Complications

23

23.1 Introduction

The gastrointestinal (GI) and hepatic systems are uniquely vulnerable to the physiological stresses of surgery and anesthesia. Postoperative GI and hepatic complications, though less frequently highlighted than cardiopulmonary issues, significantly impact recovery and outcomes.

This chapter reviews the pathophysiology, risk factors, diagnosis, and management of major postoperative GI and hepatic complications. A focus is given to postoperative jaundice, perioperative causes of hepatic dysfunction, and the historical legacy of halothane hepatitis. Postoperative nausea and vomiting (PONV), another important GI complication, is only briefly mentioned here and is discussed in detail in Chap. 25.

23.2 Postoperative GI Complications

23.2.1 Postoperative Ileus

23.2.1.1 Definition and Pathophysiology

Postoperative ileus is a transient impairment of coordinated bowel motility after surgery. It is mediated by surgical trauma, inflammatory mediators, neurohumoral changes, electrolyte disarray (e.g., hypokalemia), and perioperative opioid administration.

23.2.1.2 Risk Factors

- Abdominal and colorectal surgery
- Opioid analgesia
- Electrolyte imbalances (e.g., hypokalemia and hypomagnesemia)
- Intra-abdominal infection or peritoneal inflammation

A. Mirrakhimov, *Anesthesiology Demystified for the Internist*,
https://doi.org/10.1007/978-3-032-16811-5_23

23.2.1.3 Clinical Features and Diagnosis

Patients present with abdominal distension, delayed passage of flatus, nausea, and intolerance to oral intake. Abdominal radiographs typically show diffuse bowel dilatation without a transition point.

23.2.1.4 Management

- Bowel rest with gradual reintroduction of diet
- Minimization of opioids (multimodal or regional analgesia)
- Correction of electrolytes
- Enhanced recovery after surgery measures, such as early ambulation and chewing gum, may aid in the recovery of gut motility.

23.2.2 GI Bleeding

23.2.2.1 Etiology

- Stress ulceration in critically ill patients
- Peptic ulcer disease
- Mallory–Weiss tears from forceful vomiting
- Anastomotic bleeding
- Variceal hemorrhage in patients with cirrhosis

23.2.2.2 Management

- Stress ulcer prophylaxis (e.g., proton pump inhibitors (PPIs) and histamine 2 receptor (H2) blockers) in high-risk patients
- Endoscopic evaluation and intervention when feasible
- Transfusion support with hemoglobin and hemostatic targets
- Interventional radiology or surgical re-exploration if uncontrolled

23.2.3 Anastomotic Leak

23.2.3.1 Epidemiology and Clinical Impact

Anastomotic leaks occur in 1–5% of GI resections and are associated with increased morbidity and mortality.

23.2.3.2 Clinical Features

Fever, abdominal pain, leukocytosis, sepsis, or peritonitis. Diagnosis is confirmed with a computed tomography (CT) scan and contrast studies.

23.2.3.3 Management

- Early recognition and source control
- Broad-spectrum antibiotics
- Percutaneous or surgical drainage of fluid collections
- Reoperation for repair or diversion in severe cases

23.2.4 Mesenteric and Intestinal Ischemia

23.2.4.1 Etiology

Causes include hypotension, low cardiac output states, embolic events, or in situ thrombosis.

23.2.4.2 Clinical Features

Severe abdominal pain, lactic acidosis, hemodynamic shock (usually in the form of distributive shock), and elevated lactate dehydrogenase (LDH).

23.2.4.3 Management

- Rapid hemodynamic optimization
- Surgical or endovascular revascularization if feasible
- Resection of necrotic bowel if irreversible ischemia

23.2.5 Postoperative Nausea and Vomiting

PONV is one of the most common postoperative complications, with significant patient discomfort and potential consequences such as aspiration and wound dehiscence. It is discussed in detail in Chap. 25.

23.3 Postoperative Hepatic Complications

23.3.1 Postoperative Jaundice

23.3.1.1 Epidemiology

Postoperative jaundice occurs in up to 20% of patients, though severe cases are less common. It reflects hyperbilirubinemia due to prehepatic, hepatic, or posthepatic causes.

23.3.1.2 Etiologies

- *Prehepatic:* Hemolysis (transfusion reaction, hematoma resorption)
- *Hepatic:* Ischemic hepatitis, drug-induced injury, sepsis-associated cholestasis, and viral hepatitis
- *Posthepatic*: Biliary obstruction from gallstones, strictures, or iatrogenic bile duct injury

23.3.1.3 Diagnosis and Evaluation

- Serum bilirubin fractions
- Aspartate aminotransferase (AST)/alanine aminotransferase (ALT) versus alkaline phosphatase (ALP)/gamma-glutamyl transferase (GGT) patterns for hepatocellular versus cholestatic disease
- Ultrasound and magnetic resonance cholangiopancreatography (MRCP) for suspected obstruction

23.3.1.4 Management

- Directed therapy based on cause (optimize perfusion, treat infection, discontinue hepatotoxins, and relieve obstruction)
- Supportive monitoring of liver and renal function

23.3.2 Ischemic Hepatitis ("Shock Liver")

23.3.2.1 Pathophysiology

Occurs from global or regional hypoperfusion (shock, hypoxemia, and cardiac arrest).

23.3.2.2 Clinical Features

Aminotransferase elevations often >1000 U/L, elevated LDH, mild hyperbilirubinemia, and reversible injury if perfusion is restored promptly.

23.3.2.3 Management

- Correction of hemodynamic instability and hypoxemia
- Supportive monitoring with anticipation of resolution within days if the insult is corrected

23.3.3 Drug-Induced Liver Injury

23.3.3.1 Halothane Hepatitis

Halothane was associated with idiosyncratic, immune-mediated hepatitis, which was often severe or even fatal. Pathogenesis involved the formation of trifluoroacetyl-protein, inducing an immune response. Risk increased with repeated exposures. Incidence was estimated to be at 1 in 35,000 adults. Halothane is now largely abandoned in adult anesthesia in developed countries.

23.3.3.2 Novel Volatile Anesthetics (Isoflurane, Sevoflurane, and Desflurane)

- *Evidence*: Rare cases of hepatitis resembling halothane liver injury have been reported with modern volatile anesthetics. Case reports and small series describe hepatocellular injury with jaundice, fever, and eosinophilia (in some cases) occurring days after exposure.
- *Proposed Mechanism*: Like halothane, isoflurane, desflurane, and sevoflurane undergo oxidative metabolism by CYP2E1, producing trifluoroacetylated protein adducts, though at much lower rates than halothane. These adducts may trigger immune-mediated hepatotoxicity in genetically susceptible patients.
- *Epidemiology*: Incidence is extremely low, with most evidence limited to isolated case reports rather than large cohort studies. Compared to halothane, the risk is negligible but potentially not zero.

- *Clinical Implication*: While modern volatile anesthetics are considered safe, vigilance is warranted, especially in patients with prior volatile anesthetic-related hepatic injury.

23.3.4 Sepsis-Associated Cholestasis

Sepsis can impair bile secretion and transport, leading to conjugated hyperbilirubinemia. Cytokine-mediated downregulation of hepatocellular transport proteins plays a major role. Management requires aggressive treatment of infection and supportive care.

23.3.5 Other Perioperative Causes of Hepatic Dysfunction

- Right heart failure with hepatic congestion
- Total parenteral nutrition-associated cholestasis
- Transfusion-related hemolysis and iron overload
- Graft-versus-host disease in transplant recipients

23.4 Management Principles

- *Risk Identification*: Preoperative recognition of cirrhosis, viral hepatitis, or alcohol use
- *Optimization*: Correction of coagulopathy and careful hemodynamic management
- *Drug Stewardship*: Avoidance of unnecessary hepatotoxins
- *Monitoring*: Serial liver function tests and coagulation parameters
- *Supportive Care*: Nutritional support, infection prevention, and ICU-based organ support
- *Multidisciplinary Approach*: Early hepatology or gastroenterology consultation for severe hepatic dysfunction

23.5 Conclusion

Postoperative GI and hepatic complications remain important sources of morbidity and mortality. GI complications range from ileus to catastrophic anastomotic leaks or mesenteric ischemia. Hepatic complications include postoperative jaundice, ischemic hepatitis, drug-induced injury, and sepsis-related cholestasis. The history of halothane hepatitis underscores the importance of anesthetic-related hepatotoxicity; modern volatile agents may induce similar immune-mediated hepatitis, though such cases are exceedingly rare. Recognizing these risks, preventing complications where possible, and ensuring prompt evaluation and management are essential to improving perioperative outcomes.

Key Takeaways

1. Postoperative GI complications include ileus, bleeding, leaks, and ischemia; these must be recognized early for effective intervention.
2. Postoperative jaundice has diverse etiologies, including hemolysis, hepatocellular injury, and biliary obstruction; systematic evaluation is essential.
3. Halothane hepatitis is of historical importance, demonstrating immune-mediated anesthetic hepatotoxicity, while modern volatiles very rarely cause similar reactions.
4. Ischemic hepatitis and sepsis-associated cholestasis are common perioperative causes of hepatic dysfunction in critically ill patients.
5. Anesthesiologists play a central role in prevention, risk stratification, hemodynamic management, and multidisciplinary coordination for GI and hepatic complications.

Suggested Reading

1. Mythen MG. Postoperative gastrointestinal tract dysfunction: an overview of causes and management strategies. Cleve Clin J Med. 2009;76(Suppl 4):S66–71.
2. De la Plaza LR, Ramia JM. Postoperative complications in gastrointestinal surgery: a "hidden" basic quality indicator. World J Gastroenterol. 2019;25(23):2833–8.
3. Mazzotta E, Villalobos-Hernandez EC, Fiorda-Diaz J, et al. Postoperative ileus and postoperative gastrointestinal tract dysfunction: pathogenic mechanisms and novel treatment strategies beyond colorectal enhanced recovery after surgery protocols. Front Pharmacol. 2020;11:583422.
4. Ishii M, Mizuguchi T, Harada K, et al. Comprehensive review of post-liver resection surgical complications and a new universal classification and grading system. World J Hepatol. 2014;6(10):745–51.
5. Merath K, Tiwari A, Court C, et al. Postoperative liver failure: definitions, risk factors, prediction models and prevention strategies. J Gastrointest Surg. 2023;27(11):2640–9.
6. Habibollahi P, Mahboobi N, Esmaeili S, et al. Halothane-induced hepatitis: a forgotten issue in developing countries. Hepat Mon. 2011;11(1):3–6.
7. Nicoll A, Moore D, Njoku D, et al. Repeated exposure to modern volatile anaesthetics may cause chronic hepatitis as well as acute liver injury. BMJ Case Rep. 2012;2012:bcr2012006543.
8. LiverTox: clinical and research information on drug-induced liver injury. Desflurane. Bethesda: National Institute of Diabetes and Digestive and Kidney Diseases; 2012. Available from: https://www.ncbi.nlm.nih.gov/books/NBK548717/?utm_source=chatgpt.com.
9. Masin-Spasovska J, Dimitrovski K, Stavridis S, et al. Acute fulminant hepatatis in kidney transplant recipient after repeated sevoflurane anesthesia–a case report and literature review. Curr Drug Saf. 2013;8(2):141–4.
10. Rajan S, Garg D, Cummings KC 3rd, et al. Hepatotoxicity after sevoflurane anaesthesia: a new twist to an old story. Br J Anaesth. 2019;122(4):e63–4.
11. Cheron C, Hoet P, Renard N, et al. Fulminant hepatic failure in the course of an outpatient anesthetic procedure: sevoflurane among other high-risk factors. Case Rep Anesthesiol. 2020;2020:5124098.
12. Ryu DK, Park M, Woo S, et al. Postoperative liver injury after sevoflurane or propofol anesthesia in patients undergoing non-cardiac surgery: a retrospective cohort study. Sci Rep. 2024;14(1):11178.
13. Faust TW, Reddy KR. Postoperative jaundice. Clin Liver Dis. 2004;8(1):151–66.

Postoperative Coagulopathy and Bleeding

24

24.1 Introduction

Bleeding after surgery ranges from oozing at wound surfaces to life-threatening hemorrhage requiring re-exploration. Causes are classically divided into surgical (e.g., suboptimal surgical hemostasis) and hemostatic in cases of underlying coagulopathy. In practice, they often coexist: brisk bleeding blunts clot formation; aggressive crystalloid fluid resuscitation dilutes calcium, platelets, and coagulation factors; and hypothermia and acidosis depress enzyme kinetics. A reproducible approach is to identify surgical sources, stabilize physiology, and correct specific hemostatic defects.

24.2 Pathophysiology of Postoperative Coagulopathy

24.2.1 Hemodilution and Factor Depletion

Large-volume crystalloid/colloid (e.g., albumin) administration and cardiotomy suction, priming of cardiopulmonary bypass (CPB) in cardiac surgery with crystalloid or albumin, dilute platelets, fibrinogen, and clotting-dependent factors.

24.2.2 Hypothermia, Acidosis, and Hypocalcemia

Enzymatic coagulation is both temperature- and pH-dependent. Hypothermia (≤35 °C) reduces thrombin generation and platelet function, while acidosis (pH <7.2) impairs fibrin polymerization. Citrate in allogeneic blood products chelates calcium, further reducing coagulation factor activity. The combination of acidosis, hypothermia, and hypocalcemia—the so-called "lethal triad"—commonly coexists in massive hemorrhage and trauma.

A. Mirrakhimov, *Anesthesiology Demystified for the Internist*,
https://doi.org/10.1007/978-3-032-16811-5_24

24.2.3 Platelet Dysfunction

Quantitative loss (thrombocytopenia) and qualitative dysfunction occur after CPB (contact with artificial surfaces in the CPB circuit, hemodilution, and shear stress), in cases of uremia or advanced renal disease, hypothermia, and drugs (e.g., aspirin and P2Y12 inhibitors).

24.2.4 Coagulation Factor Dysfunction

Vitamin K-dependent factors (II, VII, IX, and X) decrease with hemodilution, liver dysfunction, in patients receiving warfarin, or malnutrition. Prolonged prothrombin time (PT)/international normalized ratio (INR) suggests deficiency of extrinsic pathway factors or warfarin effect; prolonged aPTT raises concern for intrinsic pathway defects or heparin effect.

24.2.5 Hyperfibrinolysis

Surgical tissue injury releases tissue plasminogen activator; CPB and trauma can trigger pathologic fibrinolysis with premature clot breakdown. Viscoelastic testing can identify elevated lysis, guiding antifibrinolytic therapy.

24.2.6 Disseminated Intravascular Coagulation (DIC)

Systemic procoagulant activation consumes platelets and fibrinogen and generates fibrin degradation products. Triggers include sepsis, massive tissue injury, obstetric catastrophes, and malignant disease. DIC may present as oozing plus microthrombi-related organ dysfunction.

24.2.7 Endothelial and Inflammatory Perturbations

Surgery and extracorporeal circuits disrupt endothelial glycocalyx, activate complement, and release cytokines that modulate thrombin generation, platelet function, and fibrinolysis. The net effect is context-dependent dyscrasia.

24.3 Special Contexts

24.3.1 CPB-Associated Coagulopathy

CPB causes hemodilution, hypothermia, platelet activation and depletion, contact activation, and fibrinolysis. Residual heparin or heparin rebound, as well as excessive protamine administration relative to the heparin dose, may contribute to post-protamine bleeding. Prolonged CPB or complex aortic work amplifies the hemostatic problem; antifibrinolytics (e.g., tranexamic acid) and viscoelastic-guided algorithms reduce allogenic transfusion requirements and re-exploration.

24.3.2 Massive Transfusion in the OR

Acute coagulopathy of shock and trauma is typically characterized by low fibrinogen levels, platelet dysfunction, and hyperfibrinolysis. Balanced resuscitation, early fibrinogen replacement, calcium supplementation, and the use of antifibrinolytic agents form the cornerstone of management.

24.3.3 Hepatic and Renal Dysfunction

Liver disease alters the synthesis and clearance of coagulation factors; the hemostatic system in cirrhosis is rebalanced but fragile, with both bleeding and thrombosis possible. Uremia impairs platelet adhesion and aggregation; desmopressin (DDAVP) or dialysis can transiently improve function. Drug accumulation (e.g., low molecular weight heparin (LMWH) in renal failure) can exacerbate bleeding.

24.4 Risk Stratification

Preoperative evaluation should cover:

- *Drug exposures*: Aspirin, P2Y12 inhibitors, warfarin, DOACs, heparins, selective serotonin reuptake inhibitors (SSRIs), and herbal agents (ginkgo and garlic)
- *Comorbidities*: Liver disease, renal failure, hematologic disorders (von Willebrand disease (vWD) and hemophilia), and prior bleeding
- *Surgical factors*: Anticipated blood loss, cardiac surgery with CPB use, redo sternotomy, and major spine/pelvic surgery.

Use institutional tools and specialty guidelines to pre-plan reversal windows and bridging needs, and to ensure product availability (e.g., fibrinogen concentrate, prothrombin complex concentrates, and specific antidotes).

24.5 Diagnostic Framework

24.5.1 Clinical Assessment

Differentiate surgical bleeding (bright, brisk, localized; hemodynamic instability despite adequate coagulation labs) from coagulopathic bleeding (diffuse oozing, generalized field bleeding, and persistent drain output despite hemostasis).

24.5.2 Laboratory Tests

- CBC with platelet count
- PT/INR and aPTT
- Fibrinogen (Clauss method): thresholds commonly targeted ≥150–200 mg/dL; higher targets (≥200–250 mg/dL) in cardiac surgery/obstetrics
- D-dimer, fibrin degradation products (DIC evaluation)
- Anti-Xa (heparin/LMWH effect), thrombin time (direct thrombin inhibitor effect)

Viscoelastic testing (e.g., thromboelastography (TEG) and rotational thromboelastometry (ROTEM)) provides a real-time assessment of clot formation, strength, and fibrinolysis, offering valuable insight into the underlying nature of coagulopathy (such as functional platelet deficiency, for example) and guiding targeted blood product administration. Although turnaround times have improved considerably—with results often available within an hour, these tests still represent a snapshot of prior coagulation status. Therefore, resuscitation and transfusion decisions should continue to rely primarily on ongoing hemodynamic parameters, the suspected hemorrhagic source, and the surgeon or proceduralist's assessment of hemostasis.

24.6 Management Principles

24.6.1 Step 1: Control the Source

Immediate surgical or interventional hemostasis is paramount. Re-exploration should not be delayed when clinical patterns indicate a surgical source.

24.6.2 Step 2: Correct Physiology

- *Warm the patient* (active warming to ≥36 °C).
- *Optimize pH* (treat shock, adjust ventilation, consider bicarbonate only when indicated).
- *Maintain ionized calcium* (typically ≥1.1–1.2 mmol/L) during massive transfusion (e.g., supports hemodynamics and aids in clot formation).
- *Hemodynamics*: Restore perfusion with balanced resuscitation; avoid excessive crystalloids that worsen dilutional coagulopathy.

24.6.3 Step 3: Targeted Hemostatic Therapy

24.6.3.1 Fibrinogen Repletion

- Cryoprecipitate (each unit ~150–200 mg fibrinogen) or fibrinogen concentrate for fibrinogen <150–200 mg/dL or low clot amplitude on viscoelastic testing.

24.6.3.2 Platelet Transfusion

- Transfuse for platelets <50 × 10^9/L in active bleeding (higher targets for neurosurgery/ocular surgery).
- In qualitative dysfunction (e.g., CPB, uremia, and antiplatelets), consider platelets and DDAVP.

24.6.3.3 Coagulation Factor Replacement

- *Fresh Frozen Plasma or FFP* (10–15 mL/kg) for broad factor deficiency with prolonged PT/INR and activated partial thromboplastin time (aPTT) in patients with hemorrhage
- *Prothrombin complex concentrates, aka PCC* (e.g., 25–50 IU/kg), for rapid reversal of vitamin K antagonist effect or selected factor deficiencies, faster correction, and less volume than FFP
- *Prothrombin complex versus plasma*: PCC preferred for urgent warfarin reversal in bleeding; follow with vitamin K (5–10 mg IV)

24.6.3.4 Antifibrinolytics

- *Tranexamic acid (TXA)*: useful in CPB, major orthopedic/spine, obstetric bleeding, and hyperfibrinolysis by viscoelastics. Typical dosing strategies vary by context; avoid in active intravascular clotting without bleeding.
- *Aminocaproic acid is* an alternative to TXA.

24.6.3.5 Heparin and Protamine

- If residual heparin effects are suspected (especially post-CPB), titrated protamine guided by activated clotting time (ACT) or heparin/protamine titration assays. Beware that protamine excess can cause paradoxical anticoagulation and bleeding.
- Protamine can occasionally cause hypotension during administration via multiple mechanisms, with the most severe manifestation being acute pulmonary vasoconstriction and right ventricular failure. Risk factors for protamine reactions include prior exposure (especially in diabetics using NPH insulin), fish allergy, previous vasectomy, and rapid protamine administration.

24.6.3.6 Recombinant Activated Factor VII (rFVIIa) and Activated PCC Factor Eight Inhibitor-Bypassing Activity (FEIBA)

- Rescue therapy for refractory, life-threatening bleeding after correction of pH, temperature, calcium, fibrinogen, platelets, and surgical hemostasis. Use with multidisciplinary consensus given elevated thrombosis risk (e.g., especially in patients with mechanical cardiac valves and elevated baseline prothrombotic risk).

24.6.4 Step 4: Reverse Antithrombotics

24.6.4.1 Warfarin Vitamin K Antagonist (VKA)

- *Four-factor PCC + IV vitamin K* for active bleeding; FFP if PCC unavailable.

24.6.4.2 Direct Thrombin Inhibitor (Dabigatran)

- *Idarucizumab* is used in cases of life-threatening bleeding or urgent reversal. Hemodialysis effectively removes dabigatran and may be considered in select cases; however, it typically requires placement of a large-bore central venous catheter, which carries a bleeding risk in anticoagulated patients.

24.6.4.3 Factor Xa Inhibitors (Apixaban, Rivaroxaban, and Edoxaban)

- *Andexanet alfa* for life-threatening bleeding where available; four-factor PCC as an alternative approach.

24.6.4.4 Unfractionated Heparin/LMWH

- Protamine sulfate completely reverses the anticoagulant effect of unfractionated heparin unfractionated heparin (UFH) but only partially neutralizes low-molecular-weight heparin LMWH.

24.6.4.5 Antiplatelet Agents

- *Aspirin*: Usually does not require reversal; platelet transfusion can be considered in select cases.
- *P2Y12 inhibitors*: Hold preoperatively when feasible. In the setting of urgent bleeding, platelet transfusion may be beneficial. Desmopressin can also be considered, though supporting evidence is variable. Its administration may lead to hypotension from vasodilatory effects and hyponatremia due to enhanced renal water reabsorption, necessitating close hemodynamic and electrolyte monitoring.

24.7 Massive Transfusion Protocols (MTPs)

MTPs standardize rapid delivery of red blood cells, plasma, and platelets (often in ~1:1:1 ratios) with early calcium supplementation, active warming, and laboratory/viscoelastic feedback to pivot toward factor- or fibrinogen-first strategies. Anticipated complications include hyperkalemia, hypocalcemia, hypothermia, and citrate toxicity.

Often, surgical patients develop brisk bleeding requiring rapid blood transfusion. This requires having large-bore intravenous access and a rapid infuser device. Two commercially available rapid infuser devices are shown in Fig. 24.1.

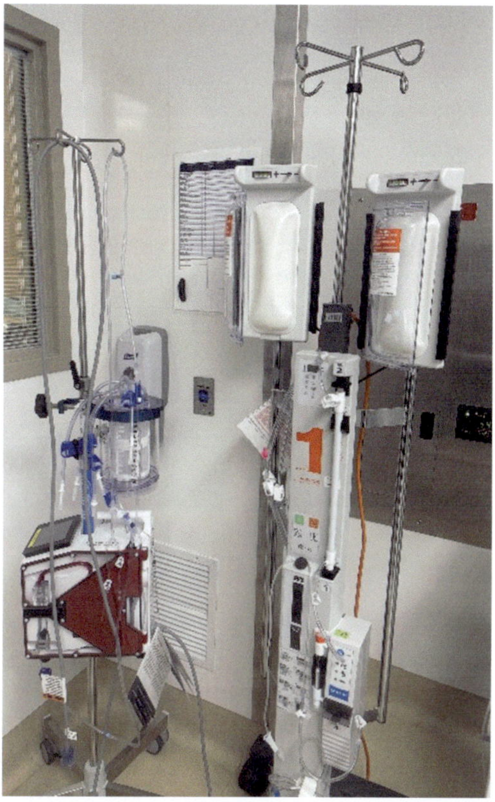

Fig. 24.1 Commercially available rapid infuser devices

24.8 Transfusion Risks and Mitigation

- *Transfusion-related Acute lung injury (TRALI)*: Acute noncardiogenic pulmonary edema within 6 hours of transfusion
- *Transfusion-associated circulatory overload (TACO)*: Volume overload; monitor net fluid balance and consider diuretics in susceptible patients
- Alloimmunization, infection risk, and immunomodulation

- To minimize these risks, particular attention should be directed toward achieving meticulous hemostasis, applying restrictive transfusion thresholds when appropriate, optimizing preoperative anemia (with iron supplementation ± erythropoiesis-stimulating agents), employing cell salvage when feasible, and using antifibrinolytics in high-risk surgical procedures.

24.8.1 Postoperative Monitoring and Re-Bleeding Prevention

- Serial hemoglobin/platelets, PT/INR, aPTT, fibrinogen, and targeted viscoelastic checks when available.
- Close surveillance for rebound anticoagulation (e.g., after protamine or PCC), late hyperfibrinolysis, and compartment syndromes.
- Maintain strict blood pressure control, as hypertension can precipitate bleeding or disrupt fragile surgical hemostasis. Patients at particular risk include those undergoing neurosurgery, vascular surgery, or cardiac surgery, as well as individuals with uncontrolled chronic hypertension.
- Early mobilization and DVT prophylaxis once hemostasis is secured, balancing bleeding risk against thromboembolic complications.

24.9 Conclusion

Postoperative coagulopathy lies at the intersection of surgical technique, physiology, and pharmacology. A structured, physiology-guided approach emphasizing rapid source control, correction of temperature, pH, and calcium, and targeted, algorithmic hemostatic therapy helps limit blood loss, reduce allogeneic transfusion requirements, and improve outcomes. The integration of viscoelastic testing within patient blood management programs, coupled with evidence-based antithrombotic reversal strategies, forms the foundation of modern perioperative care. Ultimately, success depends on early recognition, multidisciplinary coordination, and disciplined implementation of standardized protocols tailored to the surgical context.

Key Takeaways

1. Differentiate surgical from coagulopathic bleeding and address both simultaneously source control plus physiology-guided hemostatic therapy.
2. *Fix the basics first*: Temperature, pH, ionized calcium, and hemodynamics; these are foundational to effective coagulation.
3. *Targeted replacement works best*: Prioritize fibrinogen and platelets based on labs/viscoelastics; use plasma or PCC for factor deficits and TXA for hyperfibrinolysis.
4. Reverse antithrombotics promptly and specifically (PCC/Vit K for warfarin; idarucizumab for dabigatran; andexanet or PCC for Xa inhibitors; and protamine for heparins).
5. Embed care within patient blood management to minimize transfusion risks (TRALI/TACO) and improve outcomes through standardized algorithms and multidisciplinary teamwork.

Suggested Reading

1. Levy JH, Szlam F, Tanaka KA, et al. Fibrinogen and hemostasis: a primary hemostatic target for the management of acquired bleeding. Anesth Analg. 2012;114(2):261–74.
2. Kozek-Langenecker SA, Ahmed AB, Afshari A, et al. Management of severe perioperative bleeding: guidelines from the European Society of Anaesthesiology. Eur J Anaesthesiol. 2017;34(6):332–95.
3. Halme ALE, Roshanov PS, Tornberg SV, et al. Timing of major postoperative bleeding among patients undergoing surgery. JAMA Netw Open. 2024;7(4):e244581.
4. Moore EE, Moore HB, Kornblith LZ, et al. Trauma-induced coagulopathy. Nat Rev Dis Primers. 2021;7(1):30.
5. Bartoszko J, Karkouti K. Managing the coagulopathy associated with cardiopulmonary bypass. J Thromb Haemost. 2021;19(3):617–32.
6. Levy JH, Ghadimi K, Kizhakkedathu JN, et al. What's fishy about protamine? Clinical use, adverse reactions, and potential alternatives. J Thromb Haemost. 2023;21(7):1714–23.
7. Erdoes G, Faraoni D, Koster A, et al. Perioperative considerations in management of the severely bleeding coagulopathic patient. Anesthesiology. 2023;138(5):535–60.
8. White K, Faruqi U, Cohen AT. New agents for DOAC reversal: a practical management review. Br J Cardiol. 2022;29(1):1.
9. Hartmann J, Hermelin D, Levy JH. Viscoelastic testing: an illustrated review of technology and clinical applications. Res Pract Thromb Haemost. 2022;7(1):100031.

25 Postoperative Nausea and Vomiting: Risk, Prevention, and Treatment

25.1 Introduction

Nausea and vomiting are among the most feared post-anesthetic complications for patients, often ranking above pain as causes of dissatisfaction. Although often objectively benign, postoperative nausea and vomiting (PONV) can lead to serious complications, including aspiration pneumonia, electrolyte disturbances, wound dehiscence, and unanticipated need for hospital admission. This chapter explores risk assessment, prevention, and management, while emphasizing the importance of excluding other causes of PONV. Although some risk factors and management principles overlap with the pediatric population, this chapter focuses primarily on adult patients.

25.2 Epidemiology and Clinical Significance

- *Incidence*: Approximately 20–30% in general surgical populations, but up to 80% in high-risk groups
- *Impact*: Patient dissatisfaction, increased length of post-anesthesia care unit stay, unanticipated hospital admission, delayed mobilization, risk of aspiration, and wound or anastomotic complications
- *Economic Burden*: Increased costs from prolonged recovery, additional pharmacotherapy, and unplanned admissions

25.3 Pathophysiology

PONV arise from complex interactions between central and peripheral mechanisms:

- *Chemoreceptor Trigger Zone (CTZ)* in the area postrema of the medulla oblongata detects blood-borne emetogenic stimuli (e.g., opioids and anesthetics).

A. Mirrakhimov, *Anesthesiology Demystified for the Internist*,
https://doi.org/10.1007/978-3-032-16811-5_25

- *Vomiting Center* integrates inputs from the CTZ, vestibular system, GI tract, and higher cortical centers.
- *Neurotransmitters involved*: Serotonin (5-HT3), dopamine (D2), histamine (H1), acetylcholine (muscarinic), and substance P (NK1).
- *Peripheral triggers*: Mechanical gut manipulation, peritoneal irritation, and delayed gastric emptying stimulate vagal afferents.

25.4 Risk Factors

25.4.1 Patient-Related

- Female gender
- Nonsmoking status
- History of PONV or motion sickness
- Young age (<50 years)

25.4.2 Anesthesia-Related

- Use of volatile anesthetics and nitrous oxide
- Perioperative opioid administration
- Longer duration of anesthesia

25.4.3 Surgery-Related

- Procedures involving the middle ear, strabismus, laparoscopic or gynecologic surgery, and thyroid/parathyroid surgery
- Prolonged surgical duration

25.4.4 Risk Scoring

The Apfel simplified risk score assigns 1 point for each of the following: female gender, nonsmoker, history of PONV or motion sickness, and use of postoperative opioids. Risk increases from 10% (0 factors) to ~80% (four factors).

25.5 Prevention Strategies

25.5.1 General Measures

- Adequate hydration
- Avoidance of emetogenic anesthetics (e.g., volatile agents and nitrous oxide) when feasible

- Opioid-sparing multimodal analgesia (e.g., acetaminophen, non steroidal anti inflammatory drugs (NSAIDs), and regional anesthesia)
- Use of total intravenous anesthesia with propofol in high-risk patients

25.5.2 Pharmacologic Prophylaxis

Multimodal prophylaxis is recommended for patients with more than two risk factors. Common classes:

1. *Serotonin (5-HT3) antagonists (e.g., ondansetron, granisetron, and palonosetron)*
   - Mechanism: Block 5-HT3 receptors in CTZ and vagal afferents
   - Side effects: Headache, constipation, and QT prolongation
2. *Dopamine (D2) antagonists (e.g., droperidol and metoclopramide)*
   - Mechanism: Inhibit dopaminergic signaling in CTZ.
   - Side effects: Sedation, extrapyramidal symptoms, and QT prolongation. Extrapyramidal symptoms are presented in Table 25.1.
3. *Corticosteroids*
   - Mechanism: Possibly reduces serotonin release and has central antiemetic action. Dexamethasone has a delayed onset of action and therefore should be administered early, typically at the time of induction of general anesthesia.
   - Side effects: Hyperglycemia and perineal burning if given rapidly.
4. *NK1 antagonists (e.g., aprepitant and fosaprepitant)*
   - Mechanism: Block substance P at NK1 receptors in the CTZ and vomiting center
   - Side effects: Fatigue, hiccups, and drug–drug interactions
5. *Anticholinergics (e.g., scopolamine patch)*
   - Mechanism: Block muscarinic receptors in vestibular pathways. It has a delayed onset of action and should therefore be applied early, typically in the preoperative period. Patients with glaucoma should avoid its use, and all patients should be counseled to wash their hands after patch removal, as residual medication can cause transient blurred vision if inadvertently transferred to the eyes.
   - Side effects: Dry mouth, blurred vision, urinary retention, and confusion in the elderly.

Table 25.1 Summary of extrapyramidal reactions

Syndrome	Clinical presentation	Treatment
Tardive dyskinesia	Involuntary choreoathetoid movements (e.g., face, tongue, and limbs)	Stop the medication. Benzodiazepines. Psychiatry consultation.
Akathisia	Urge to move, restlessness	Stop the medication. Propranolol and benztropine may be considered.
Parkinsonism	Masked facies, cogwheel rigidity, tremor, and bradykinesia	Stop the medication. Benztropine, diphenhydramine may be considered. Neurology consultation.
Acute dystonia	Involuntary contraction of a muscle group	Stop the medication. Benztropine, diphenhydramine may be considered.

6. *Antihistamines (e.g., dimenhydrinate and diphenhydramine)*
   - Mechanism: H1 receptor antagonism, especially useful in vestibular nausea
   - Side effects: Sedation and anticholinergic effects

25.5.3 Timing of Prophylaxis

- Dexamethasone: at induction
- 5-HT3 antagonists: at the end of surgery
- NK1 antagonists: preoperatively due to slower onset
- Scopolamine patch: applied preoperatively

25.6 Acute Treatment

1. *Exclude alternative diagnoses*:
   - Acute pancreatitis: epigastric pain and elevated lipase
   - Inferior wall myocardial infarction (MI): nausea, vomiting, bradycardia, and ST segment changes on the 12 lead electrocardiogram
   - Bowel obstruction
   - Cholelithiasis and hepatobiliary pathology
   - Acute appendicitis
2. *Rescue Therapy*
   - Choose an agent from a different class than used for prophylaxis if appropriate.
   - Examples:
     - If prophylaxis was ondansetron + dexamethasone, consider droperidol or promethazine for rescue if not contraindicated.
     - If no prophylaxis was administered, ondansetron is often the first-line.
3. *Non-Pharmacologic Adjuncts*
   - Acupuncture/acupressure.
   - Inhalation of isopropyl alcohol vapors has been shown to help alleviate PONV.
   - Adequate hydration.

25.7 Special Considerations

25.7.1 Ambulatory and Outpatient Surgery

PONV are a major cause of delayed discharge and unanticipated admission. Prophylaxis is particularly important in these patients.

Table 25.2 Mechanisms and side effects of common medications used in PONV prevention and treatment

Drug class	Mechanism	Common side effects
5-HT3 antagonists	Block serotonin at CTZ/vagal afferents	Headache, QT interval prolongation, constipation
Dopamine antagonists	Block D2 in CTZ	Sedation, extrapyramidal symptoms, QT interval prolongation
Corticosteroids	Modulate serotonin/neurokinin pathways	Hyperglycemia, perineal burning
NK1 antagonists	Block substance P/NK1	Fatigue, hiccups, CYP3A4 interactions
Anticholinergics	Block muscarinic receptors	Dry mouth, confusion, urinary retention
Antihistamines	Block H1	Sedation, anticholinergic effects

25.7.2 High-Risk Populations

- Women undergoing gynecologic or breast surgery
- Patients with prior severe PONV
- Patients requiring opioids despite multimodal analgesia

A summary of medications used in the prevention and treatment of PONV is presented in Table 25.2.

25.8 Conclusion

PONV remain a common and distressing postoperative complication, but one that is largely preventable and treatable through structured risk assessment, multimodal prophylaxis, and evidence-based acute treatment. Awareness of risk factors and pharmacologic mechanisms is key to successful prophylaxis and therapy. Clinicians must also remain vigilant for alternative diagnoses that can mimic PONV but require urgent intervention, such as acute myocardial infarction or pancreatitis. Effective prevention and management of PONV not only enhances patient satisfaction but also reduces complications, improves efficiency, and decreases healthcare utilization.

Key Takeaways

1. PONV are common, affecting up to 80% of high-risk patients, and significantly impact recovery and satisfaction.
2. Risk factors include female sex, nonsmoking status, prior PONV/motion sickness, opioids, volatile agents, and specific surgeries.
3. Prevention is most effective when based on risk stratification and multimodal prophylaxis with different drug classes.
4. Acute management requires ruling out alternative diagnoses and selecting rescue therapy from a different mechanistic class.
5. Understanding the mechanism and side effects of antiemetics allows safe, effective, and tailored PONV management.

Suggested Reading

1. Apfel CC, Laara E, Koivuranta M, et al. A simplified risk score for predicting PONV. Anesthesiology. 1999;91(3):693–700.
2. Gan TJ, Diemunsch P, Habib AS, et al. Consensus guidelines for the management of PONV. Anesth Analg. 2014;118(1):85–113.
3. Jin Z, Gan TJ, Bergese SD. Prevention and treatment of postoperative nausea and vomiting (PONV): a review of current recommendations and emerging therapies. Ther Clin Risk Manag. 2020;16:1305–17.
4. Weibel S, Rücker G, Eberhart LH, et al. Drugs for preventing PONV in adults after general anesthesia: a network meta-analysis. Cochrane Database Syst Rev. 2017;11:CD012859.
5. Zhang Z, Wang X. The neural mechanism and pathways underlying postoperative nausea and vomiting: a comprehensive review. Eur J Med Res. 2025;30(1):362.
6. Kovac AL. Pathophysiology and risk factors for postoperative nausea and vomiting in adults and children. BJA Educ. 2025;25(6):234–9.

Malignant Hyperthermia: Pathophysiology, Diagnosis, Prevention, and Management

26

26.1 Introduction

Malignant hyperthermia (MH) remains one of the most feared anesthesia complications, owing to its explosive onset, severity of metabolic derangements, and potential lethality. Understanding its pathogenesis, recognition, and management is vital for anesthesiologists and perioperative clinicians. Equally important is differentiating MH from conditions with overlapping features, such as exertional rhabdomyolysis and muscular dystrophies, that require distinct management strategies.

26.2 Etiology and Pathogenesis

26.2.1 Genetic Basis of MH

- Autosomal dominant inheritance with variable penetrance.
- Most cases are linked to RYR1 mutations; less commonly, calcium voltage-gated channel subunit alpha 1S (CACNA1S) mutations.
- Abnormal channels permit excessive calcium efflux when exposed to triggering agents.

26.2.2 Cellular Mechanism

- *Normal physiology*: Membrane depolarization opens dihydropyridine receptors, activating RyR1 to release calcium from the sarcoplasmic reticulum.
- *MH-susceptible physiology*: Triggers cause uncontrolled calcium release, leading to sustained contraction, adenosine triphosphate (ATP) depletion, excessive heat generation, lactic acidosis, hypercarbia, and rhabdomyolysis.

A. Mirrakhimov, *Anesthesiology Demystified for the Internist*,
https://doi.org/10.1007/978-3-032-16811-5_26

26.3 Risk Factors and Susceptible Conditions

26.3.1 Definite Risks

- Family or personal history of MH.
- Known RYR1 or CACNA1S mutations.
- Congenital myopathies are strongly associated with MH (e.g., central core disease, multi-minicore disease, and King-Denborough syndrome).
- Exposure to triggers: all volatile anesthetics (see Fig. 26.1) and succinylcholine (see Fig. 26.2). Nitrous oxide is not considered a triggering agent for MH.

26.3.2 Exertional Rhabdomyolysis

Exertional rhabdomyolysis can mimic some features of MH and has been linked in rare cases to underlying RYR1 genetic variants. While not all patients with exertional rhabdomyolysis are MH-susceptible, some overlap exists. Patients with recurrent or severe exertional rhabdomyolysis may merit evaluation in a specialized MH center, particularly if genetic or biopsy evidence of RyR1 abnormality is found.

26.3.3 Duchenne and Becker Muscular Dystrophy

- These dystrophinopathies are not associated with MH.
- However, succinylcholine and volatile anesthetics may cause severe, rapid-onset hyperkalemia and rhabdomyolysis, often leading to ventricular arrhythmia and cardiac arrest.
- Therefore, these agents should be strictly avoided, and alternative anesthesia (e.g., total intravenous anesthesia (TIVA) with propofol, opioids, and nondepolarizing relaxants) should be used.

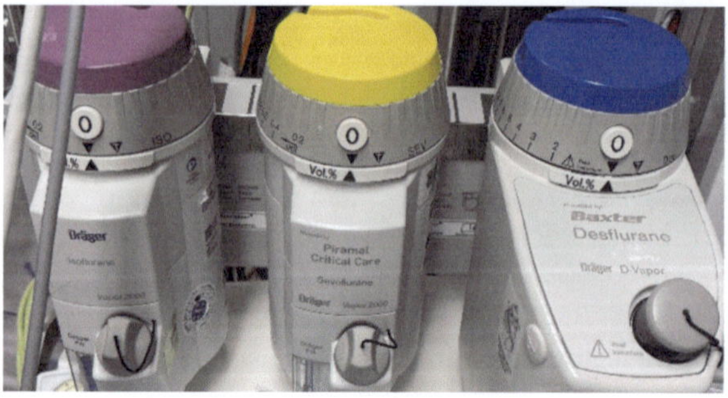

Fig. 26.1 Volatile anesthetics attached to an anesthesia machine

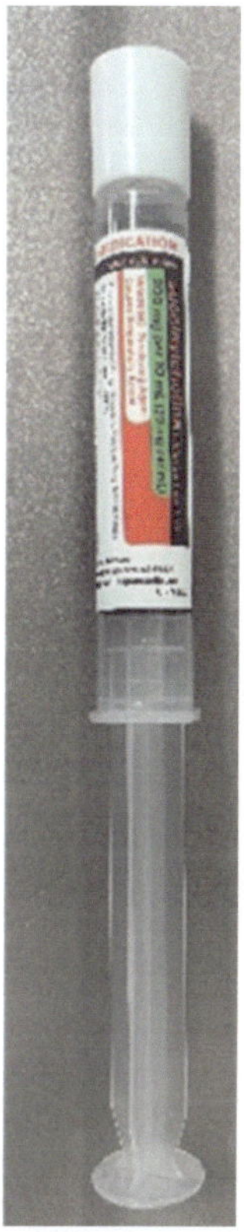

Fig. 26.2 Succinylcholine syringe

26.3.4 Demographics of MH

- Male predominance, higher frequency in children and young adults.
- MH can occur at any age if susceptible.

26.4 Clinical Presentation

26.4.1 Early Signs

- Rapid, unexplained rise in end-tidal CO_2 (despite increased ventilation)
- Tachycardia (often the earliest cardiovascular clue)
- Generalized or masseter rigidity, especially after succinylcholine
- Labored or rapid breathing and hypertension

26.4.2 Progressive Features

- Hyperthermia (>1 °C increase every 5 min; late finding)
- Mixed metabolic and respiratory acidosis
- Hyperkalemia with arrhythmias
- Myoglobinuria and dark urine
- Disseminated intravascular coagulation in severe cases

26.4.3 Timing and Fever Considerations

- MH usually arises intraoperatively or within 1 hour after anesthesia.
- Fever developing >1 hour post-anesthesia is unlikely to be MH and should prompt evaluation for alternative diagnoses such as sepsis, transfusion reaction, thyroid storm, or neuroleptic malignant syndrome.

26.5 Diagnosis

26.5.1 Clinical

- Diagnosis is clinical and urgent. Treatment should not be delayed for confirmatory testing.

26.5.2 Monitoring and Laboratory Findings Supporting MH

- *Capnography*: rapid end tidal carbon ($ETCO_2$) rise
- *Arterial blood gas*: acidosis
- *Labs*: hyperkalemia, elevated creatine kinase (CK) (often >10,000 U/L), myoglobinemia, myoglobinuria, and acute kidney injury
- *Electocardiogram (ECG)*: peaked T waves and arrhythmias

26.5.3 Definitive Testing

This testing is not available at the time of the suspected reaction and should be performed only after the acute episode has been fully managed and the patient has stabilized.

- *Caffeine-halothane contracture test*: Gold standard.
- *Genetic testing*: Genetic testing can identify pathogenic variants in RYR1 or CACNA1S; however, negative results do not fully exclude MH susceptibility, as not all causative mutations have been discovered or are available for testing.

26.6 Prevention

26.6.1 Preoperative Assessment

- Careful family and personal history of anesthesia complications, rhabdomyolysis, or muscle disease
- Genetic counseling and testing when suspicion is high

26.6.2 Anesthetic Planning

- Avoid triggering agents (e.g., volatile agents and succinylcholine).
- Employ strict TIVA (propofol, opioids, and non-depolarizing neuromuscular blockers).
- Anesthesia machine preparation: Remove vaporizers (which deliver volatile anesthetics to the patient), flush the anesthesia machine with high fresh gas flows, and apply activated charcoal filters to adsorb any residual anesthetic vapors.
- Ensure dantrolene availability in all facilities using triggering anesthetic agents.

26.7 Management

26.7.1 Immediate Actions

1. Stop triggering agents immediately. Apply activated charcoal filters to the anesthesia machine to adsorb any remaining volatile anesthetics.
2. Call for help.
3. *Call the Malignant Hyperthermia Association of the United States for guidance at 1-800-644-9737 (available 24/7).*
4. *Administer dantrolene sodium* (commercially available as Ryanodex®, requiring fewer vials and rapid reconstitution, and as Revonto® or Dantrium®, which require multiple vials and larger fluid volumes). Initial dose: 2.5 mg/kg IV, repeat as needed up to 10 mg/kg. Continue 1 mg/kg every 4–6 h or as continuous infusion for 24–48 h.

26.7.2 Supportive Therapy

- *Hyperventilation with 100% oxygen.*
- *Active cooling*: IV cold saline, surface cooling, gastric/bladder lavage until <38 °C.
- *Correct acidosis*: sodium bicarbonate if pH <7.2.
- *Manage hyperkalemia*: insulin/glucose, IV calcium (but avoid using calcium channel blockers together with dantrolene because the combination can cause

life-threatening cardiovascular collapse, hyperkalemia, and myocardial depression), beta-agonists, and hemodialysis if needed.
- *Treat arrhythmias* with agents other than calcium channel blockers.
- *Maintain urine output* (mannitol, furosemide, and fluids).

26.7.3 Post-Crisis Care

- ICU monitoring for 24–48 hours for risk of recrudescence.
- Monitor for renal failure, compartment syndrome, electrolyte abnormalities, and disseminated intravascular coagulation.

26.8 Differential Diagnosis

- Sepsis
- Thyroid storm
- Neuroleptic malignant syndrome
- Serotonin syndrome
- Pheochromocytoma crisis
- Heat stroke
- Acute cocaine/amphetamine intoxication
- Anaphylaxis

26.9 Prognosis

- With the advent and routine use of dantrolene, the mortality of MH has declined to less than 5%.
- Delayed diagnosis and inadequate treatment increase the risk of multiorgan failure and death.
- Survivors should be referred for MH testing and genetic counseling.

26.10 Conclusion

MH is a pharmacogenetic hypermetabolic crisis triggered by volatile anesthetics and succinylcholine in susceptible patients. Recognition of early signs such as unexplained hypercapnia and rigidity is critical, since hyperthermia is usually a late manifestation. Dantrolene and supportive measures dramatically reduce mortality. Patients with exertional rhabdomyolysis may overlap genetically with MH and warrant careful preoperative evaluation, though not all are at truly increased risk.

Patients with Duchenne and Becker muscular dystrophy are not MH susceptible but are vulnerable to catastrophic hyperkalemia when exposed to succinylcholine and volatile anesthetics; hence, these agents are avoided. Finally, postoperative fever appearing more than 1 h after anesthesia is very unlikely to represent MH and should prompt alternative diagnostic considerations.

Key Takeaways
1. MH is a pharmacogenetic disorder of calcium regulation triggered by volatile anesthetics and succinylcholine.
2. Exertional rhabdomyolysis may share genetic overlap with MH in some individuals, but not all are at increased risk.
3. Duchenne and Becker muscular dystrophy are not MH risks but predispose to fatal hyperkalemia with succinylcholine and volatiles.
4. Early recognition (rise in $ETCO_2$, rigidity, and tachycardia) and dantrolene administration are life-saving.
5. Fever >1 h after anesthesia is unlikely MH, and alternative diagnoses should be sought.

Suggested Reading

1. Rosenberg H, Pollock N, Schiemann A, et al. Malignant hyperthermia: a review. Orphanet J Rare Dis. 2015;10:93.
2. Pinyavat T, Riazi S, Deng J, et al. Malignant hyperthermia. Crit Care Med. 2024;52(12):1934–40.
3. Glahn KP, Ellis FR, Halsall PJ, et al. Recognizing and managing a malignant hyperthermia crisis: guidelines from the European Malignant Hyperthermia Group. Br J Anaesth. 2010;105(4):417–20.
4. Halsall PJ, Robinson RL. Malignant hyperthermia and associated conditions. Handb Clin Neurol. 2007;86:107–24.
5. Hopkins PM. Malignant hyperthermia: pharmacology of triggering. Br J Anaesth. 2011;107(1):48–56.
6. Souliere CR Jr, Weintraub SJ, Kirchner JC. Markedly delayed postoperative malignant hyperthermia. Arch Otolaryngol Head Neck Surg. 1986;112(5):564–6.
7. Litman RS, Flood CD, Kaplan RF, et al. Postoperative malignant hyperthermia: an analysis of cases from the North American Malignant Hyperthermia Registry. Anesthesiology. 2008;109(5):825–9.
8. Min JY, Hong SH, Kim SJ, et al. Delayed-onset malignant hyperthermia in the postanesthetic care unit: a case report. J Int Med Res. 2021;49(9):3000605211044201.
9. Barnes C, Stowell KM, Bulger T, et al. Safe duration of postoperative monitoring for malignant hyperthermia patients administered non-triggering anaesthesia: an update. Anaesth Intensive Care. 2015;43(1):98–104.
10. Rüffert H, Bastian B, Bendixen D, et al. Consensus guidelines on perioperative management of malignant hyperthermia suspected or susceptible patients from the European Malignant Hyperthermia Group. Br J Anaesth. 2021;126(1):120–30.

Local Anesthetic Systemic Toxicity: Recognition, Prevention, and Management

27

27.1 Introduction

Local anesthetics (LAs) are central to modern perioperative and pain management practice. They are used in peripheral nerve blocks, neuraxial anesthesia, infiltration techniques, and perineural catheters for continuous analgesia. Although considered safe, accidental intravascular injection or excessive systemic absorption can lead to LA systemic toxicity (LAST). Historically, LAST carried high morbidity and mortality, but advances in prevention, early recognition, and lipid emulsion therapy have improved survival. This chapter reviews the etiology, pathogenesis, risk factors, prevention, and management of LAST with special consideration of novel formulations and advanced rescue strategies.

27.2 Etiology and Pathogenesis

27.2.1 Mechanisms of LAST

- *Direct intravascular injection*: Most dangerous mechanism; can cause immediate seizures or cardiac collapse.
- *Systemic absorption from block site*: Gradual accumulation occurs in highly vascular regions (e.g., intercostal, paravertebral, and truncal blocks) or with excessive total dose.
- *Excessive dosing*: Ignoring maximum recommended limits significantly increases risk. Safe dosing of LAs is summarized in Table 27.1. Reported values may vary slightly depending on the reference source. Importantly, these recommendations are not derived from robust evidence, and clinical variability exists: some patients may develop LAST despite receiving doses within the recommended range, whereas others may tolerate seemingly excessive doses without toxicity. Nonetheless, the published dosing guidelines should be used as the standard when calculating the maximum allowable dose of LAs.

A. Mirrakhimov, *Anesthesiology Demystified for the Internist*,
https://doi.org/10.1007/978-3-032-16811-5_27

Table 27.1 Recommended dosing of LAs

Agent	Max dose (without epinephrine)	Max dose (with epinephrine)	Comments
Lidocaine	4.5 mg/kg	7 mg/kg	Widely used; low cardiotoxicity
Mepivacaine	5 mg/kg	7 mg/kg	Intermediate duration
Ropivacaine	3 mg/kg	3.5 mg/kg	Less cardiotoxic than bupivacaine
Bupivacaine	2.5 mg/kg	3 mg/kg	Most cardiotoxic; avoid overdose

27.2.2 Pharmacology of Toxicity (The Reader Is Referred to Chap. 12 for More Information)

- At therapeutic levels, LAs stabilize neuronal membranes by blocking voltage-gated sodium channels.
- At toxic levels, this extends to the central nervous system (CNS) and cardiovascular system:
  - *CNS*: Excitation → seizures → depression → coma/respiratory arrest.
  - *Cardiac*: Conduction block, negative inotropy, ventricular arrhythmias, and cardiovascular collapse.
- *Bupivacaine* is especially cardiotoxic because it binds sodium channels tightly and dissociates slowly, complicating resuscitation.

27.3 Risk Factors

27.3.1 Patient-Related

- Extremes of age (neonates and elderly)
- Frailty or low muscle mass
- Hepatic/renal dysfunction (impaired metabolism/clearance)
- Cardiac disease or limited reserve
- Pregnancy (increased sensitivity and decreased protein binding)

27.3.2 Procedure-Related

- *Truncal/fascial plane blocks*: Large volumes of LA and increased tissue vascularity enhance systemic absorption.
- *Perineural catheters*: Continuous or intermittent bolus infusions can lead to gradual accumulation and delayed toxicity; vigilance with dosing and monitoring is required.
- Large-volume infiltration or bilateral blocks

Epinephrine decreases systemic absorption, prolongs the duration of action, and acts as a marker for inadvertent intravascular injection.

27.4 Liposomal Bupivacaine

- Multivesicular liposome formulation allows sustained release up to 96 hours.
- *Benefits*: Potential for prolonged analgesia (controversial), opioid-sparing.
- *Risks*: LAST can still occur if overdosed or injected intravascularly.
- *Guideline*: Do not administer additional LAs for 96 hours after liposomal bupivacaine due to additive toxicity via increase in cumulative plasma bupivacaine levels.

27.5 Clinical Presentation

27.5.1 Neurologic

- Typically, neurologic symptoms appear first: tinnitus, perioral numbness, metallic taste, agitation, and confusion.
- Progression may include seizures, altered consciousness, coma, and respiratory arrest.

27.5.2 Cardiovascular

- In most patients, cardiac toxicity follows neurologic symptoms.
- However, in some cases—particularly with potent and highly cardiotoxic agents such as bupivacaine—cardiac manifestations may be the presenting feature, including conduction block, ventricular arrhythmias, severe bradycardia, or sudden cardiovascular collapse without preceding CNS signs.

27.6 Prevention

1. Adhere to maximum safe doses.
2. Add epinephrine to LA (marker of intravascular injection and reduced uptake).
3. Incremental injection with frequent aspiration.
4. Ultrasound guidance (reduces but does not eliminate risk).
5. Avoid rapid bolus of large volumes.
6. Adjust dosing in neonates, elderly, pregnant, or patients with comorbidities.
7. Ensure immediate availability of resuscitation equipment and lipid emulsion.

27.7 Management

27.7.1 Immediate Actions

- Immediately discontinue LA administration, including any ongoing continuous infusions (e.g., perineural catheter or epidural)
- Call for help and activate LAST protocol.

- Secure airway and administer 100% O_2.
- Treat seizures with benzodiazepines (avoid large doses of propofol).

27.7.2 Lipid Emulsion Therapy (See Fig. 27.1)

- *Bolus*: 1.5 mL/kg 20% lipid emulsion IV over 1 minute
- *Infusion*: 0.25 mL/kg/min; increase to 0.5 mL/kg/min if unstable.
- *Repeat bolus* as needed
- *Max dose*: ~10–12 mL/kg in the first 30 min

27.7.3 Circulatory Support

- *Epinephrine*: Small doses (<1 mcg/kg). Large doses may impair resuscitation and worsen acidosis.
- *Avoid vasopressin*: May increase pulmonary vascular resistance and worsen acidosis in the setting of LAST.

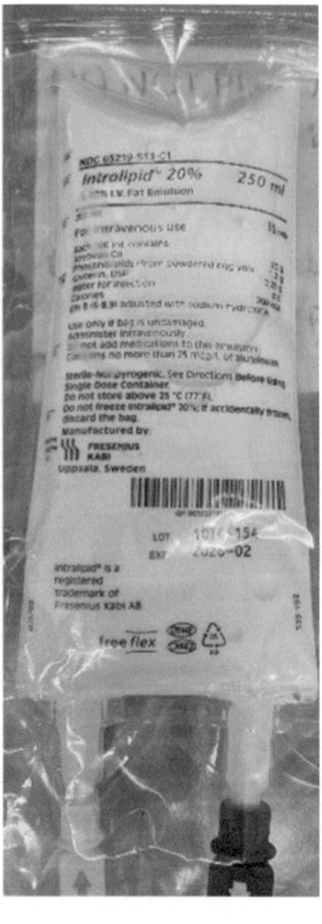

Fig. 27.1 Commercially available lipid emulsion bag for intravenous administration

- *Avoid calcium channel blockers and beta-blockers*: Carry a potential to exacerbate myocardial depression and conduction abnormalities in the setting of LAST.
- It is important to note that the recommendation to avoid vasopressin, calcium channel blockers, and beta-blockers during LAST management is supported primarily by animal studies, case reports, and mechanistic concerns, rather than randomized controlled human trials.
- *Amiodarone* is preferred for ventricular arrhythmias. Intravenous lidocaine should not be used to treat ventricular arrhythmias in the setting of LAST, as it is itself an LA and may exacerbate toxicity.

27.7.4 Advanced Rescue

- *Extracorporeal membrane oxygenation (ECMO) or cardiopulmonary bypass (CPB)*: In refractory cases with cardiovascular collapse unresponsive to conventional therapy and lipid rescue, ECMO or CPB provides circulatory support until the toxin redistributes and is metabolized. Access to these modalities may be limited, but early consideration is recommended for centers with the capability.

27.7.5 Post-Crisis Care

- ICU admission for 12–24 hours monitoring (longer if severe).
- Monitor for recurrence due to redistribution.
- Watch for renal injury from rhabdomyolysis.

27.8 Conclusion

LAST is a rare but potentially catastrophic complication. It can result from inadvertent intravascular injection, excessive systemic dosing and absorption, or cumulative dosing with continuous perineural catheters. Bupivacaine is the most cardiotoxic LA, whereas liposomal bupivacaine carries unique risks, necessitating avoidance of additional LAs for at least 96 h after administration. Prevention relies on careful dosing, incremental injection, epinephrine use, and ultrasound guidance. Management requires rapid recognition, seizure control, airway support, and early lipid emulsion therapy. Small epinephrine doses are useful for resuscitation, while vasopressin, calcium channel blockers, and beta-blockers should be avoided. ECMO and CPB can be lifesaving in refractory LAST when conventional measures fail.

Key Takeaways

1. LAST is most often due to intravascular injection or excessive absorption, especially during truncal blocks or continuous infusions.
2. Bupivacaine is the most cardiotoxic LA; liposomal formulations require strict avoidance of additional LAs for 96 hours.

3. Prevention includes safe dosing, epinephrine, incremental injection, and ultrasound guidance.
4. Management centers on airway support, seizure control, lipid emulsion therapy, and cautious circulatory support (small epinephrine doses).
5. Refractory cases may require ECMO or CPB for survival until drug redistribution.

Suggested Reading

1. Macfarlane AJR, Gitman M, Bornstein KJ, et al. Updates in our understanding of local anaesthetic systemic toxicity: a narrative review. Anaesthesia. 2021;76(Suppl 1):27–39.
2. Gitman M, Fettiplace MR, Weinberg GL, et al. Local anesthetic systemic toxicity: a narrative literature review and clinical update on prevention, diagnosis, and management. Plast Reconstr Surg. 2019;144(3):783–95.
3. Fettiplace MR, Weinberg G. The mechanisms underlying lipid resuscitation therapy. Reg Anesth Pain Med. 2018;43(2):138–49.
4. Barrington MJ, Kluger R. Ultrasound guidance reduces the risk of local anesthetic systemic toxicity following peripheral nerve blockade. Reg Anesth Pain Med. 2013;38(4):289–99.
5. Bacon B, Silverton N, Katz M, et al. Local anesthetic systemic toxicity induced cardiac arrest after topicalization for transesophageal echocardiography and subsequent treatment with extracorporeal cardiopulmonary resuscitation. J Cardiothorac Vasc Anesth. 2018;33(1):162–5.
6. Ilfeld BM, Sessler DI. Liposomal bupivacaine in peripheral nerve blocks: duration and meaningful differences. Anesthesiology. 2024;141(4):638–42.
7. Hamilton TW, Athanassoglou V, Mellon S, Strickland LH, Murray D. Liposomal bupivacaine infiltration at the surgical site for the management of postoperative pain. Cochrane Database Syst Rev. 2017;2:CD011419.
8. Belfar AL, Nguyen PN, Feng BH. Local anaesthetic systemic toxicity presenting as cardiac arrest after subcutaneous infiltration of liposomal bupivacaine. Br J Anaesth. 2025;135(1):232–3.
9. https://www.nysora.com/topics/complications/local-anesthetic-systemic-toxicity/.

28 Postoperative Pain Management

28.1 Introduction

Postoperative pain is not only a symptom but a risk factor for complications and prolonged post-surgical recovery. Untreated pain impairs effective breathing and ventilation, coughing, and mobilization, leading to atelectasis, pneumonia, and thromboembolic events. Inadequate control also predisposes to chronic post-surgical pain and increased opioid dependence. The reader is referred to Chap. 12 for more information.

The goals of perioperative pain management are to:

1. Provide effective analgesia to enable early mobilization and rehabilitation.
2. Minimize opioid-related side effects and long-term dependence.
3. Tailor approaches for special populations, including those with chronic pain and opioid use disorders.
4. Employ multimodal strategies to leverage synergistic analgesic effects.

28.2 Pathophysiology of Postoperative Pain

Surgical pain is a complex interplay of nociceptive, inflammatory, and sometimes neuropathic mechanisms:

- *Nociceptive pain*: Tissue injury activates nociceptors.
- *Inflammatory pain*: Release of prostaglandins, bradykinin, and cytokines sensitizes nociceptors.
- *Neuropathic pain*: Nerve injury may contribute, especially in thoracotomy, mastectomy, or limb amputations.

A. Mirrakhimov, *Anesthesiology Demystified for the Internist*,
https://doi.org/10.1007/978-3-032-16811-5_28

- *Central sensitization*: Amplification of pain signals in the central nervous system (CNS) contributes to hyperalgesia and chronic pain risk.

Understanding these mechanisms supports the rationale for multimodal analgesia, targeting multiple pathways simultaneously.

28.3 Multimodal Analgesia

28.3.1 Non-opioid Pharmacologic Options

- *Acetaminophen*: Effective baseline analgesic, opioid-sparing, safe when dosed appropriately.
- *Non steroidal anti inflammatory drugs (NSAIDs)/cyclooxygenase (COX)-2 inhibitors*: Analgesics with opioid-sparing effects; use with caution in renal impairment, bleeding risk, or cardiovascular disease.
- *Gabapentinoids (gabapentin and pregabalin)*: Can be helpful in cases of neuropathic pain and high-risk surgeries; risks include sedation and dizziness.
- *Ketamine*: Low-dose infusions reduce opioid requirements and provide antihyperalgesic effects, especially in opioid-tolerant patients.
- *Dexmedetomidine and clonidine*: Provide analgesic and sedative effects through $\alpha 2$ agonism; reduce opioid requirements but may cause bradycardia or hypotension.
- *IV lidocaine infusion*: May reduce pain and postoperative ileus in abdominal surgery, but requires monitoring due to the potential risk of local anesthetic systemic toxicity (please see Chap. 27 for more information).

28.3.2 Regional and Neuraxial Analgesia

- *Peripheral nerve blocks*: Single-shot or catheter infusions for site-specific analgesia (e.g., femoral, adductor canal, paravertebral, and brachial plexus).
- *Fascial plane blocks*: Transversus abdominis plane, erector spinae, and rectus sheath blocks are increasingly used for abdominal and thoracic procedures.
- *Epidural analgesia*: Gold standard for thoracic and major abdominal surgery, particularly effective for visceral pain.

28.3.3 Rescue Regional Techniques

When systemic analgesics are inadequate, rescue blocks or catheter placements can improve postoperative pain control, avoid opioid escalation, and improve recovery. Close collaboration with acute pain and regional anesthesia teams is essential.

28.4 Patients with Chronic Pain and Opioid Therapy

28.4.1 Patients on Buprenorphine

- *Mechanism*: Partial μ-agonist, κ-antagonist, and high receptor affinity.
- *Challenges*: Its high receptor affinity can blunt the effect of full agonist opioids.
- *Perioperative strategies*:
  - Continue buprenorphine perioperatively for most patients.
  - Supplement with multimodal analgesia, and if necessary, administer higher doses of full opioid agonists to achieve adequate pain control.
  - Consider split dosing of buprenorphine to improve analgesia.
  - Coordinate with the acute pain medicine service and addiction medicine.

28.4.2 Patients on Methadone

- *Mechanism*: Full μ-agonist with long half-life; also an M-methyl-D-aspartate (NMDA) antagonist.
- *Perioperative considerations*:
  - Continue daily methadone to prevent withdrawal.
  - Additional opioids are often required for surgical pain due to tolerance.
  - Monitor QTc interval prolongation on electrocardiogram and drug interactions.

28.4.3 Patients Using Illicit Opioids

- Present with tolerance, dependence, or withdrawal risk.
- Usually require higher opioid doses and aggressive multimodal strategies.
- Risk of relapse or diversion requires multidisciplinary management, ideally involving addiction specialists.
- Careful discharge planning and linkage to treatment programs are essential.

28.5 Opioid Stewardship

28.5.1 Principles

- Prescribe opioids only, when necessary, at the lowest effective dose, and for the shortest possible duration.
- Employ multimodal analgesia to minimize opioid needs.
- Educate patients about safe use, storage, and disposal.
- Avoid overprescription at discharge—base prescriptions on inpatient use.

28.5.2 Hospital Programs

- Enhanced recovery after surgery pathways standardize multimodal regimens.
- Audit and feedback improve prescribing patterns.
- Acute pain services provide tailored, patient-specific oversight.

28.6 Special Considerations

- *Elderly*: More sensitive to sedatives and opioids; prioritize non-opioid modalities.
- *Renal/hepatic dysfunction*: Adjust drug selection and dosing.
- *Obstructive sleep apnea*: Increased risk of opioid-induced respiratory depression; avoid long-acting opioids, and emphasize regional techniques.

28.7 Prevention of Chronic Post-Surgical Pain

- Aggressive perioperative pain control reduces the risk of central sensitization.
- Regional anesthesia and multimodal analgesia may reduce chronic pain incidence.

28.8 Conclusion

Postoperative pain management requires a comprehensive, individualized approach that emphasizes multimodal analgesia, judicious opioid use, and consideration of patient-specific factors. Patients with chronic pain, opioid maintenance therapy, or illicit opioid use present unique challenges, requiring multidisciplinary collaboration and coordination with addiction services. Rescue regional anesthesia techniques provide powerful tools to manage refractory pain while minimizing opioid burden. Opioid stewardship programs are essential to balance effective pain relief with the need to mitigate long-term dependence and societal harm.

Key Takeaways

1. Multimodal analgesia is the foundation of postoperative pain management, reducing opioid requirements and improving outcomes.
2. Patients on buprenorphine or methadone should continue therapy perioperatively, with additional multimodal and opioid support as needed.
3. Patients with illicit opioid use require higher doses and close multidisciplinary care, with addiction services involvement.
4. Rescue regional techniques are valuable for refractory pain, avoiding excessive opioid escalation.
5. Opioid stewardship is critical to reduce misuse, chronic dependence, and societal opioid burden.

Suggested Reading

1. Gordon DB, de Leon-Casasola OA, Wu CL, et al. Research gaps in practice guidelines for acute postoperative pain management in adults: findings from a review of the evidence for an American Pain Society Clinical Practice Guideline. J Pain. 2016;17(2):158–66.
2. Chou R, Gordon DB, de Leon-Casasola OA, et al. Management of postoperative pain: a clinical practice guideline from the American Pain Society, the American Society of Regional Anesthesia and Pain Medicine, and the American Society of Anesthesiologists' Committee on Regional Anesthesia, Executive Committee, and Administrative Council. J Pain. 2016;17(2):131–57.
3. Wu CL, Raja SN. Treatment of acute postoperative pain. Lancet. 2011;377(9784):2215–25.
4. Soffin EM, Lee BH, Kumar KK, et al. The prescription opioid crisis: role of the anaesthesiologist in reducing opioid use and misuse. Br J Anaesth. 2019;122(6):e198–208.
5. Alford DP, Compton P, Samet JH. Acute pain management for patients receiving maintenance methadone or buprenorphine therapy. Ann Intern Med. 2006;144(2):127–34.
6. Kohan L, Potru S, Barreveld AM, et al. Buprenorphine management in the perioperative period: educational review and recommendations from a multisociety expert panel. Reg Anesth Pain Med. 2021;46(10):840–59.
7. Goel A, Azargive S, Lamba W, et al. Perioperative considerations in patients on buprenorphine: a narrative review. Can J Anaesth. 2019;66(2):201–17.
8. Wick EC, Grant MC, Wu CL. Postoperative multimodal analgesia pain management with nonopioid analgesics and techniques. JAMA Surg. 2017;152(7):691–7.
9. Cornett EM, Kline RJ, Robichaux SL, et al. Comprehensive perioperative management considerations in patients taking methadone. Curr Pain Headache Rep. 2019;23(7):49.
10. Vadeghani AT, Grant M, Forget P. Perioperative pain management interventions in opioid user patients: an overview of reviews. BMC Anesthesiol. 2024;24(1):310.
11. Pirie K, Traer E, Finniss D, et al. Current approaches to acute postoperative pain management after major abdominal surgery: a narrative review and future directions. Br J Anaesth. 2022;129(3):378–93.

Part VI

Putting It All Together

Perioperative Consultation: Building an Effective Co-management Model

29

29.1 Introduction

As surgical populations grow older and more medically complex, the role of perioperative consultation has expanded. Traditionally, models separated preoperative evaluation, which were often mischaracterized as "clearance" (a term better replaced with "optimization" and risk stratification), typically led by internal medicine, from intraoperative and immediate postoperative care, which was the responsibility of anesthesiology. However, this siloed approach can miss opportunities for proactive risk mitigation and coordinated care. Instead, perioperative consultation is best conceptualized as a continuum of co-management, where internal medicine and anesthesiology work in partnership with surgery, nursing, and other disciplines to optimize patients' outcomes.

29.2 The Rationale for a Co-management Model

- *Increasing complexity of patients*: High prevalence of cardiovascular disease, diabetes mellitus, chronic kidney disease, and frailty is associated with perioperative risk.
- *Expansion of surgical procedures*: More patients undergo advanced surgeries, including minimally invasive approaches with complex perioperative implications.
- *Need for continuity*: Internal medicine provides longitudinal care, while anesthesiology ensures acute perioperative safety. Integration ensures that neither perspective is lost.
- *Improved outcomes with collaboration*: Studies have shown that perioperative co-management reduces complications, shortens length of stay, and improves resource utilization.

A. Mirrakhimov, *Anesthesiology Demystified for the Internist*,
https://doi.org/10.1007/978-3-032-16811-5_29

29.3 Roles and Strengths of Internal Medicine

29.3.1 Preoperative Evaluation

- Comprehensive history and physical examination
- Identification and optimization of comorbidities (e.g., hypertension, coronary artery disease, chronic obstructive pulmonary disease (COPD), chronic kidney disease (CKD), diabetes mellitus, etc.)
- Risk stratification using validated tools and models
- Medication reconciliation and perioperative management of anticoagulants, antiplatelets, and chronic therapies (e.g., beta-blockers, angiotensin converting enzyme (ACE) inhibitors, and insulin)

29.3.2 Intraoperative Consultation (As Needed)

- Provide relevant medical background to the anesthesia team.
- Offer input on unusual metabolic, endocrine, or hematologic issues.

29.3.3 Postoperative Management

- Co-management of medical complications (e.g., delirium, pneumonia, myocardial infarction (MI), arrhythmia, acute kidney injury (AKI), etc.).
- Continuity of chronic disease management.
- Transition planning back to outpatient care.

29.4 Roles and Strengths of Anesthesiology

29.4.1 Preoperative

- Focused assessment of airway, anesthetic risk, and functional capacity
- Tailoring anesthetic techniques to patient comorbidities, surgical requirements, and individual clinical nuances
- Planning perioperative monitoring and hemodynamic goals

29.4.2 Intraoperative

- Expertise in physiology under surgical stress: managing ventilation, circulation, fluid balance, and anesthesia depth
- Acute crisis management (e.g., arrhythmias, hypotension, hypoxemia, etc.).
- Coordination with the surgical team to reduce blood loss and prevent complications

29.4.3 Postoperative

- Pain management through multimodal regimens and regional techniques
- Initial hemodynamic stabilization in post operative care unit (PACU) or intensive care unit (ICU)
- Early recognition of anesthetic-related complications

29.5 Principles of Effective Co-management

29.5.1 Shared Assessment and Risk Stratification

- Combining internal medicine and anesthesiology expertise enhances the accuracy of perioperative risk prediction.
- Collaboration ensures both long-term disease implications and intraoperative stress responses are addressed.

29.5.2 Optimization of Comorbidities

- Internal medicine leads chronic disease optimization.
- Anesthesiology advises on intraoperative tolerances (e.g., safe hemodynamic targets in severe aortic stenosis, etc.).
- Joint planning for high-risk interventions (e.g., bridging anticoagulation, fluid management in patients with congestive heart failure, etc.).

29.5.3 Communication and Handoffs

- Structured communication frameworks to reduce errors.
- Joint preoperative clinics facilitate integrated planning.
- Clear postoperative handoffs between PACU, wards, and ICU ensure continuity.

29.5.4 Enhanced Recovery After Surgery

- Internal medicine supports comorbidity optimization and early mobilization.
- Anesthesiology implements multimodal and opioid sparing analgesia.
- Shared responsibility reduces complications and accelerates discharge.

29.6 Models of Co-management

1. *Consultative model*: Internal medicine provides recommendations; anesthesiology manages anesthesia independently. May lead to gaps if communication is poor.

2. *Integrated preoperative clinic*: Internal medicine and anesthesia evaluate patients jointly, providing unified risk assessment and optimization plans.
3. *Perioperative surgical home*: A comprehensive, anesthesiology-led model that incorporates principles of internal medicine for preoperative disease optimization.
4. *Co-management teams on wards*: Internal medicine and anesthesia jointly manage complex postoperative patients, particularly in orthopedics, cardiac, and transplant services.

29.7 Barriers to Effective Co-management

- *Cultural differences*: Internal medicine and anesthesiology may view perioperative care and risk differently.
- *Workflow misalignment*: Different schedules and documentation systems often hinder integration.
- *Resource limitations*: Joint clinics and dedicated staff require institutional support.
- *Role ambiguity*: Unclear responsibilities can create duplication or missed care.

29.8 Enablers of Success

- Institutional recognition of the value of co-management
- Shared electronic health records with standardized templates
- Interdisciplinary education and case conferences
- Clear leadership structures and defined roles
- Mutual respect and understanding of complementary expertise

29.9 Case Example: High-Risk Patient Undergoing Colon Resection

- Internal medicine identifies poorly controlled diabetes, chronic kidney disease, and coronary artery disease. Initiates optimization with cardiology and endocrinology as needed.
- Anesthesiology evaluates the patient's limited functional capacity, recommends invasive hemodynamic monitoring, and plans epidural analgesia to attenuate the surgical stress response, optimize postoperative pain control, and reduce reliance on rescue systemic opioids.
- Joint plan ensures perioperative beta-blockade, glucose control, fluid restriction, and early ICU admission.
- Outcome: Improved stability, reduced complications, and smoother discharge planning.

29.10 Future Directions

- Wider implementation of perioperative surgical homes
- Expanded use of digital risk prediction and decision support
- Greater integration of acute pain and chronic disease management services
- Research into patient-centered outcomes such as satisfaction, functional recovery, and quality of life

29.11 Conclusion

Perioperative consultation should be viewed not as a bureaucratic "clearance," but as a co-management model that integrates the complementary strengths of internal medicine and anesthesiology to ensure comprehensive medical optimization of complex patients before surgery. Collaborative risk assessment, comorbidity optimization, clear communication, and coordinated postoperative co-management improve outcomes, reduce complications, and enhance both patient safety and satisfaction. Building an effective model requires institutional commitment, clear role definition, and a culture of interprofessional collaboration.

Key Takeaways

1. Perioperative consultation is most effective when approached as a co-management model focused on optimizing complex patients and improving perioperative outcomes, rather than as a transactional "clearance" process.
2. Internal medicine and anesthesiology provide complementary strengths, enhancing risk stratification, optimization, and crisis management.
3. Communication and structured handoffs are essential to avoid gaps and duplication of care.
4. Enhanced recovery pathways benefit from joint ownership, combining chronic disease management and intraoperative expertise.
5. Institutional support and culture of collaboration are vital to sustain effective perioperative co-management models.

Suggested Reading

1. Thompson A, Fleischmann KE, Smilowitz NR, et al. 2024 AHA/ACC/ACS/ASNC/HRS/SCA/SCCT/SCMR/SVM guideline for perioperative cardiovascular management for noncardiac surgery: a report of the American College of Cardiology/American Heart Association Joint Committee on Clinical Practice Guidelines. Circulation. 2024;150(19):e351–442.
2. Bello C, Rössler J, Shehata P, et al. Perioperative strategies to reduce risk of myocardial injury after non-cardiac surgery (MINS): a narrative review. J Clin Anesth. 2023;87:111106.
3. Park LJ, Borges FK, Ofori S, et al. Association between complications and death within 30 days after general surgery: a vascular events in noncardiac surgery patients cohort evaluation (VISION) substudy. Ann Surg. 2025;282(6):1007–13. https://doi.org/10.1097/SLA.0000000000006372.

4. Devereaux PJ, Sessler DI. Cardiac complications in patients undergoing major noncardiac surgery. N Engl J Med. 2015;373(23):2258–69.
5. Vetter TR, Boudreaux AM, Jones KA, et al. The Perioperative Surgical Home: how anesthesiology can collaboratively achieve and leverage the triple aim in health care. Anesth Analg. 2014;118(5):1131–6.
6. Vetter TR. Managing a perioperative medicine program. Best Pract Res Clin Anaesthesiol. 2022;36(2):283–98.
7. Adesanya AO, Joshi GP. Hospitalists and anesthesiologists as perioperative physicians: are their roles complementary? Proc (Bayl Univ Med Cent). 2007;20(2):140–2.
8. Lee A, Kerridge RK, Chui PT, et al. Perioperative systems as a quality model of perioperative medicine and surgical care. Health Policy. 2011;102(2–3):214–22.
9. Khambaty M, Devalapalli AP, Silbert RE, et al. Practice changing updates in perioperative medicine literature 2022. A systematic review. Am J Med. 2023;136(8):753–62.

30 Perioperative Medicine Case Discussions: An Anesthesiologist's Perspective for Internists

30.1 Introduction

The perioperative period is inherently interdisciplinary. Internists and hospitalists play an essential role in optimizing chronic medical conditions, risk-stratifying patients, and guiding perioperative medication management. Anesthesiologists integrate this information into the dynamic intraoperative environment, where moment-to-moment physiological changes, airway control, surgical positioning, and technical considerations dictate the safest anesthetic technique.

While consultants may occasionally recommend a "preferred anesthetic technique," this can inadvertently encroach on anesthesiology's domain, as anesthetic planning requires integration of surgical needs, patient physiology, and intraoperative contingencies. Rather than prescribing an anesthesia modality, consultants should emphasize risk communication. Anesthesiologists can then operationalize these principles within a feasible and safe anesthetic plan.

The following three case-based discussions illustrate this principle. These case-based discussions do not describe any specific patient but rather summarize real-world clinical experiences. Any resemblance to actual individuals is purely coincidental.

30.2 Case 1: Severe Aortic Stenosis and Hip Fracture Surgery

30.2.1 Clinical Scenario

A 67-year-old male with severe aortic stenosis (a mean pressure gradient of 52 mm Hg and an aortic valve area of 0.9 cm^2 on transthoracic echocardiography), hypertension (on metoprolol and lisinopril), and atrial fibrillation on apixaban presents for urgent left femoral head fracture surgery after a fall. The hospital medicine consultation note recommended spinal anesthesia to avoid the "risk" of general anesthesia.

A. Mirrakhimov, *Anesthesiology Demystified for the Internist*,
https://doi.org/10.1007/978-3-032-16811-5_30

30.2.2 Considerations

30.2.2.1 Risks of General Anesthesia in Severe Aortic Stenosis (AS)

- Hemodynamic instability during induction/intubation (risk of hypotension and tachycardia)
- Risk of myocardial ischemia due to reduced coronary perfusion during hypotension
- Potential for prolonged postoperative mechanical ventilation

30.2.2.2 Risks of Spinal Anesthesia in Severe AS

- *Abrupt sympathetic blockade* → precipitous hypotension and loss of preload/afterload, which is poorly tolerated in patients with severe aortic stenosis.
- *Anticoagulation*: The patient is on apixaban; spinal anesthesia carries a significant risk of spinal/epidural hematoma.
- *Duration*: Spinal anesthesia may not last long enough for prolonged orthopedic surgery, requiring conversion to general anesthesia (GA) under urgent and suboptimal conditions.
- *Positioning and access*: Intraoperative positioning (lateral or difficult access to the airway) can complicate airway management if emergent conversion is required.

30.2.3 Why General Anesthesia Is Preferred

- Provides secure airway control throughout a long orthopedic procedure.
- Facilitates careful titration of hemodynamics with invasive monitoring (arterial line and vasopressors).
- Avoids the risk of spinal hematoma from anticoagulation.
- Prevents abrupt sympathectomy and catastrophic hypotension.

Conclusion In this patient, general anesthesia with invasive monitoring (arterial line) is safer than spinal. Regional blocks (e.g., femoral or fascia iliaca) can enhance postoperative analgesia but are insufficient to provide surgical anesthesia for this procedure on their own.

30.3 Case 2: Severe Chronic Obstructive Pulmonary Disease (COPD) and Proximal Humerus Surgery

30.3.1 Clinical Scenario

A 63-year-old female with tobacco use disorder and severe COPD (on 3 L of supplemental oxygen at baseline) presents for proximal humerus fracture repair. Hospital medicine consultation recommended surgery under nerve block to avoid general anesthesia.

30.3.2 Considerations

30.3.2.1 Surgical and Positioning Factors

- Shoulder surgery is commonly performed in the beach chair position, which limits airway access intraoperatively.
- Surgical anesthesia for shoulder surgery typically requires an interscalene block, which produces near-universal phrenic nerve paralysis, leading to a 25–30% reduction in forced expiratory volume in 1 second (FEV_1).
- In severe COPD, even small reductions in diaphragmatic function may precipitate respiratory failure.

30.3.2.2 Risks of Nerve Block as Sole Technique

- An interscalene block can provide anesthesia, but tolerance is limited by respiratory status.
- Alternative blocks (e.g., suprascapular and axillary nerve blocks) are phrenic-sparing but inadequate for surgical anesthesia, serving best as adjuncts for postoperative analgesia.
- Airway access in the beach chair position poses significant challenges should conversion to general anesthesia become necessary.

30.3.3 Why General Anesthesia Is Preferred

- Provides a secure airway with an endotracheal tube during beach chair positioning.
- Prevents hypoventilation from diaphragmatic paralysis.
- Allows for control of oxygenation/ventilation in a fragile patient with advanced respiratory disease.
- Regional techniques (suprascapular/axillary block) can still be added postoperatively for analgesia, minimizing opioid use.

Conclusion GA with airway control is safer, with adjunct nerve blocks for pain relief.

30.4 Case 3: End Stage Renal Disease (ESRD), Anxiety, and Aortic Valve (AV) Fistula Creation

30.4.1 Clinical Scenario

A 57-year-old female with poorly controlled diabetes (HbA1c 10), uncontrolled hypertension, severe anxiety/claustrophobia, and ESRD on hemodialysis (via tunneled catheter) presents for AV fistula creation. Internal medicine consultation recommended regional anesthesia to avoid GA.

30.4.2 Considerations

30.4.2.1 Risks of Regional Anesthesia Alone

- Although regional (e.g., brachial plexus block) can provide both excellent surgical anesthesia and postoperative analgesia, this patient's severe anxiety and claustrophobia make cooperation challenging.
- Inability to remain still compromises patient safety and surgical precision.
- Sedation may be inadequate, and oversedation risks airway compromise.

30.4.2.2 Benefits of General Anesthesia with Regional Block

- GA ensures immobility and safety.
- Regional block pre-induction provides analgesia, reduces intraoperative anesthetic requirements, and improves postoperative pain control.
- Regional vasodilation secondary to a brachial plexus nerve block for this patient may also enhance fistula patency and maturation.
- Close fluid/electrolyte monitoring under GA mitigates ESRD-related risks.

Conclusion GA supplemented with a regional block is safest and most effective in this anxious, high-risk patient. Analgesic regional anesthesia techniques may improve postoperative pain control and may also facilitate arteriovenous fistula maturation by inducing local sympathectomy–mediated vasodilation, thereby increasing regional blood flow.

30.5 Preoperative Internal Medicine Consultation: Focus on Optimization, Not Modality

- Internists should provide risk-focused guidance.
- Consultant recommendations on the preferred anesthetic techniques should generally be avoided, as intraoperative factors (e.g., airway access, surgical positioning, pharmacology, and monitoring) are complex and dynamic.
- Effective collaboration requires respectful communication of risks and shared goals, while leaving the anesthetic technique decision to anesthesiologists.

30.6 Conclusion

Perioperative care of complex patients demands collaboration, not competition. Internal medicine brings expertise in optimization, risk assessment, and longitudinal care. Anesthesiology applies expertise in physiology, airway management, and intraoperative decision-making. When internists suggest anesthetic techniques without considering intraoperative realities, conflicts can arise. Through respectful dialogue, shared understanding of roles, and focusing on patient-centered goals, perioperative teams can achieve safer outcomes.

These three case-based scenarios highlight how anesthesiologists integrate medical, surgical, and technical factors to choose the safest anesthetic plan. Internists should avoid recommending a specific mode of anesthesia, instead providing risk-based guidance that allows anesthesiologists to craft the appropriate plan. This co-management approach fosters trust, prevents miscommunication, and most importantly, protects the patient.

Key Takeaways
1. Perioperative anesthetic planning is complex and integrates surgical needs, patient-specific nuances, positioning, and airway considerations.
2. Spinal anesthesia poses risks in patients with severe aortic stenosis.
3. Interscalene blocks are poorly tolerated in patients with severe COPD (including other causes of advanced respiratory disease) due to phrenic nerve paralysis; GA with airway control plus phrenic-sparing blocks for analgesia should be considered.
4. Regional anesthesia alone may fail in patients with severe anxiety and claustrophobia.
5. Internists should focus on optimization and risk communication, not recommending anesthetic modality, to support anesthesiology's intraoperative expertise.

Suggested Reading

1. Tabrizi NS, Demos RA, Schumann R, et al. Neuraxial anesthesia in patients with aortic stenosis: a systematic review. J Cardiothorac Vasc Anesth. 2024;38(2):505–16.
2. Kopp SL, Vandermeulen E, McBane RD, et al. Regional anesthesia in the patient receiving antithrombotic or thrombolytic therapy: American Society of Regional Anesthesia and Pain Medicine Evidence-Based Guidelines (fifth edition). Reg Anesth Pain Med. 2025:rapm-2024-105766. https://doi.org/10.1136/rapm-2024-105766.
3. Tran DQH, Elgueta MF, Aliste J, et al. Diaphragm-sparing nerve blocks for shoulder surgery. Reg Anesth Pain Med. 2017;42(1):32–8.
4. Kang RA, Ko JS. Recent updates on interscalene brachial plexus block for shoulder surgery. Anesth Pain Med (Seoul). 2023;18(1):5–10.
5. Wang J, Hou X, Zhang X, et al. Comparison of pulmonary function during interscalene block vs. supraclavicular block: a single-center, double-blind, randomized trial. BMC Anesthesiol. 2023;23:12.
6. Jorgensen MS, Farres H, James BLW, et al. The role of regional versus general anesthesia on arteriovenous fistula and graft outcomes: a single-institution experience and literature review. Ann Vasc Surg. 2020;62:287–94.
7. Li X, Zhou Q, Zhang X, et al. Anesthesia management of a patient with claustrophobia undergoing surgery for rhegmatogenous retinal detachment: a case report. Medicine (Baltimore). 2023;102(42):e35624.

Future Directions: Perioperative Medicine as a Collaborative Specialty

31

31.1 Introduction

The practice of perioperative medicine has undergone a paradigm shift in recent decades. Once viewed narrowly as "anesthetic clearance" or intraoperative monitoring, it is now appreciated as a continuum of care requiring coordination before, during, and after surgery. This transformation reflects the realities of an aging population, rising rates of cardiovascular and metabolic disease, and the need to address long-term functional outcomes.

Internists are indispensable partners in this domain. Their skill in managing multimorbidity, optimizing chronic disease, and ensuring continuity of care complements anesthesiologists' acute intraoperative expertise. The result is a richer, more comprehensive model of perioperative medicine that aligns with the broader goals of patient-centered care, quality improvement, and value-based healthcare.

31.2 The Expanding Scope of Perioperative Medicine

31.2.1 From Clearance to Optimization

Historically, perioperative evaluation was often described as "medical clearance," a term implying binary approval for surgery. Modern practice reframes this process as risk assessment and optimization, recognizing that nearly all patients can proceed to surgery with appropriate preparation.

A. Mirrakhimov, *Anesthesiology Demystified for the Internist*,
https://doi.org/10.1007/978-3-032-16811-5_31

31.2.2 Beyond the Operating Room

Perioperative medicine now spans:

- *Preoperative phase*: Disease optimization, patient education, and medication management
- *Intraoperative phase*: Anesthetic planning, physiology control, and acute crisis management
- *Postoperative phase*: Complication prevention, enhanced recovery, pain management, and transition to home or rehabilitation

31.2.3 Multimorbidity and Complexity

The prevalence of multimorbidity, patients with chronic conditions, is steadily rising. Internists' expertise in navigating these complexities makes them essential partners in surgical planning and perioperative care.

31.3 Collaborative Models of Perioperative Care

31.3.1 Perioperative Surgical Home (PSH)

- A patient-centered, anesthesiology-led model integrating internists, surgeons, and allied professionals.
- Emphasizes continuity across the surgical journey.
- Evidence shows reduced length of stay, improved satisfaction, and decreased complications.

31.3.2 Enhanced Recovery After Surgery (ERAS)

- Protocol-driven, multidisciplinary approach aimed at reducing stress response, accelerating mobilization, and minimizing opioid use.
- Requires integration of anesthesiology (fluid management and pain control), internal medicine (chronic disease optimization), and surgery (minimally invasive techniques).

31.3.3 Co-management Models

- Joint inpatient management between internal medicine and surgical/anesthesia teams
- Proven to reduce complications and readmissions in high-risk surgeries (e.g., orthopedic and vascular)

31.4 Innovations Shaping the Future

31.4.1 Digital Health and Predictive Analytics

- Machine learning models and artificial intelligence to aid in the prediction of perioperative risk of complications (e.g., acute kidney injury (AKI), myocardial infarction (MI), and readmission)
- Wearable devices and telemedicine for prehabilitation and postoperative monitoring

31.4.2 Patient-Centered Outcomes

- Greater emphasis on functional recovery, quality of life, and patient-reported outcomes
- Shift from "survival alone" to "recovery with function"

31.4.3 Opioid Stewardship and Pain Pathways

- Multimodal analgesia, regional techniques, and enhanced pain services to reduce opioid exposure and chronic dependence
- Close partnership with internal medicine in managing patients with chronic opioid use or substance use disorders

31.4.4 Expanding Role of Hospitalists

- Hospitalists increasingly co-lead perioperative programs, given their expertise in inpatient medicine, multidisciplinary coordination, and systems-based practice

31.5 Barriers and Challenges

- *Resource limitations*: Building perioperative clinics and co-management teams requires institutional support and investment.
- *Cultural silos*: Overcoming historical divisions between specialties requires deliberate collaboration.
- *Role clarity*: Defining responsibilities prevents duplication or gaps in care.
- *Education*: Training curricula must evolve to incorporate perioperative medicine across both internal medicine and anesthesiology.

31.6 The Essential Role of Internists in Perioperative Care

Internists are uniquely positioned to:

- Optimize patients with complex comorbidities prior to surgery.
- Provide nuanced medication management (e.g., anticoagulation, antihypertensives, diabetes therapy, etc.).
- Manage postoperative complications such as delirium, sepsis, or acute coronary events.
- Ensure smooth transitions from surgical admission back to outpatient follow-up.

Their presence ensures that perioperative medicine remains connected to the broader arc of chronic disease care, rather than a discrete hospital episode.

31.7 Conclusion

Perioperative medicine is entering a new era: one defined by integration, innovation, and collaboration. Internists and anesthesiologists must work together to optimize outcomes for increasingly complex surgical patients. The future is not about delineating boundaries but about building bridges. In this vision, perioperative medicine becomes not just a phase of care, but a model of interprofessional excellence that exemplifies the very best of modern medicine.

Key Takeaways

1. Perioperative medicine is evolving into a collaborative field, uniting internal medicine, anesthesiology, surgery, and allied health.
2. Internists play an essential role in chronic disease optimization, risk stratification, and continuity, anchoring perioperative care in long-term patient health.
3. Collaborative models such as ERAS, PSH, and co-management reduce complications and improve patient-centered outcomes.
4. Future directions emphasize innovation: predictive analytics, digital health, functional outcomes, and opioid stewardship.
5. Interdisciplinary collaboration is the foundation of safe, effective, and patient-centered perioperative care.

Suggested Reading

1. Vetter TR, Boudreaux AM, Jones KA, et al. The perioperative surgical home: how anesthesiology can collaboratively achieve and leverage the triple aim. Anesth Analg. 2014;118(5):1131–6.
2. Stier G, Ramsingh D, Raval R, et al. Anesthesiologists as perioperative hospitalists and outcomes in patients undergoing major urologic surgery: a historical prospective, comparative effectiveness study. Perioper Med (Lond). 2018;7:13.

3. Bryan YF, Kolarzyck L. From ship captains to crew members in a history of relationships between anesthesiologists and surgeons. AMA J Ethics. 2020;22(4):E333–9.
4. Ron D, Gunn CM, Havidich JE, et al. Preoperative communication between anesthesia, surgery, and primary care providers for older surgical patients. Jt Comm J Qual Patient Saf. 2024;50(5):326–37.
5. Gharapetian A, Chung F, Wong D, et al. Perioperative fellowship curricula in anesthesiology: a systematic review. Can J Anaesth. 2015;62(4):403–12.
6. Thompson RE, Pfeifer K, Grant PJ, et al. Hospital medicine and perioperative care: a framework for high-quality, high-value collaborative care. J Hosp Med. 2017;12(4):277–82.

Epilogue: A Personal Journey From Medical Optimization to Intraoperative Management

32

When I first trained in internal medicine, I thought I had a solid understanding of perioperative care. I could rattle off the Revised Cardiac Risk Index, adjust beta-blockers, and issue the ever-popular (and usually vague) recommendation: *"Avoid hypotension."* What more could anesthesiology possibly need from me?

Then I crossed into anesthesiology.

As a new trainee in the operating room, I realized just how little I truly knew about the nuances of this field. It wasn't just about keeping a patient "asleep"; it was about moment-to-moment physiology, airway strategy in extremely challenging circumstances, resuscitation in the setting of active hemorrhage, and orchestrating medications with time courses so short they could be measured in heartbeats. Suddenly, the phrase *"avoid hypotension"* seemed almost comically insufficient. It was a bit like telling a pilot, "Just don't crash" before a transatlantic flight.

This dual training gave me a rare perspective: I learned the value of each discipline not only in its own domain but also in the way it complements the other. Internal medicine grounds perioperative care in the patient's lifelong health journey, such as comorbidities, medication use, and chronic disease trajectories. Anesthesiology manages the acute storm of surgery and invasive procedures, steering physiology through controlled chaos with vigilance and precision. Neither can succeed in isolation; both need each other.

So, when I stress throughout this book that internists should focus on optimization and risk communication and leave anesthetic technique to the anesthesiologists, it comes from a place of lived experience in both specialties. I know the temptation to "recommend spinal" or "avoid general anesthesia," because I once made those very suggestions myself. And I also know the quiet smile that spreads across an anesthesiologist's face when they hear it, the smile that says, "If only you knew what I know."

The future of perioperative medicine is not about whose specialty leads, but how we co-lead. It is about trust, respect, and partnership. Internists must continue to anchor surgical care in the broader arc of patient health, and anesthesiologists must

A. Mirrakhimov, *Anesthesiology Demystified for the Internist*,
https://doi.org/10.1007/978-3-032-16811-5_32

continue to navigate the acute intraoperative storm. Together, we form a team greater than the sum of its parts.

If this book has given you a new appreciation for that collaboration, if it makes you pause before writing "clear for surgery" and instead think in terms of optimization, communication, and partnership, then it has done its job.

And if it also made you smile at my early missteps, all the better. After all, perioperative medicine is serious work—but it works best when we approach it together, with humility, curiosity, and just the right dose of humor, titrated to effect.

—From someone who once thought anesthesia was just "pushing propofol and solving sudoku."

Index

A. Mirrakhimov, *Anesthesiology Demystified for the Internist*,
https://doi.org/10.1007/978-3-032-16811-5

O

P

Q

R

MIX
Papier aus verantwortungsvollen Quellen
Paper from responsible sources
FSC® C105338

If you have any concerns about our products,
you can contact us on
ProductSafety@springernature.com

In case Publisher is established outside the EU,
the EU authorized representative is:
Springer Nature Customer Service Center GmbH
Europaplatz 3, 69115 Heidelberg, Germany

Printed by Libri Plureos GmbH
in Hamburg, Germany